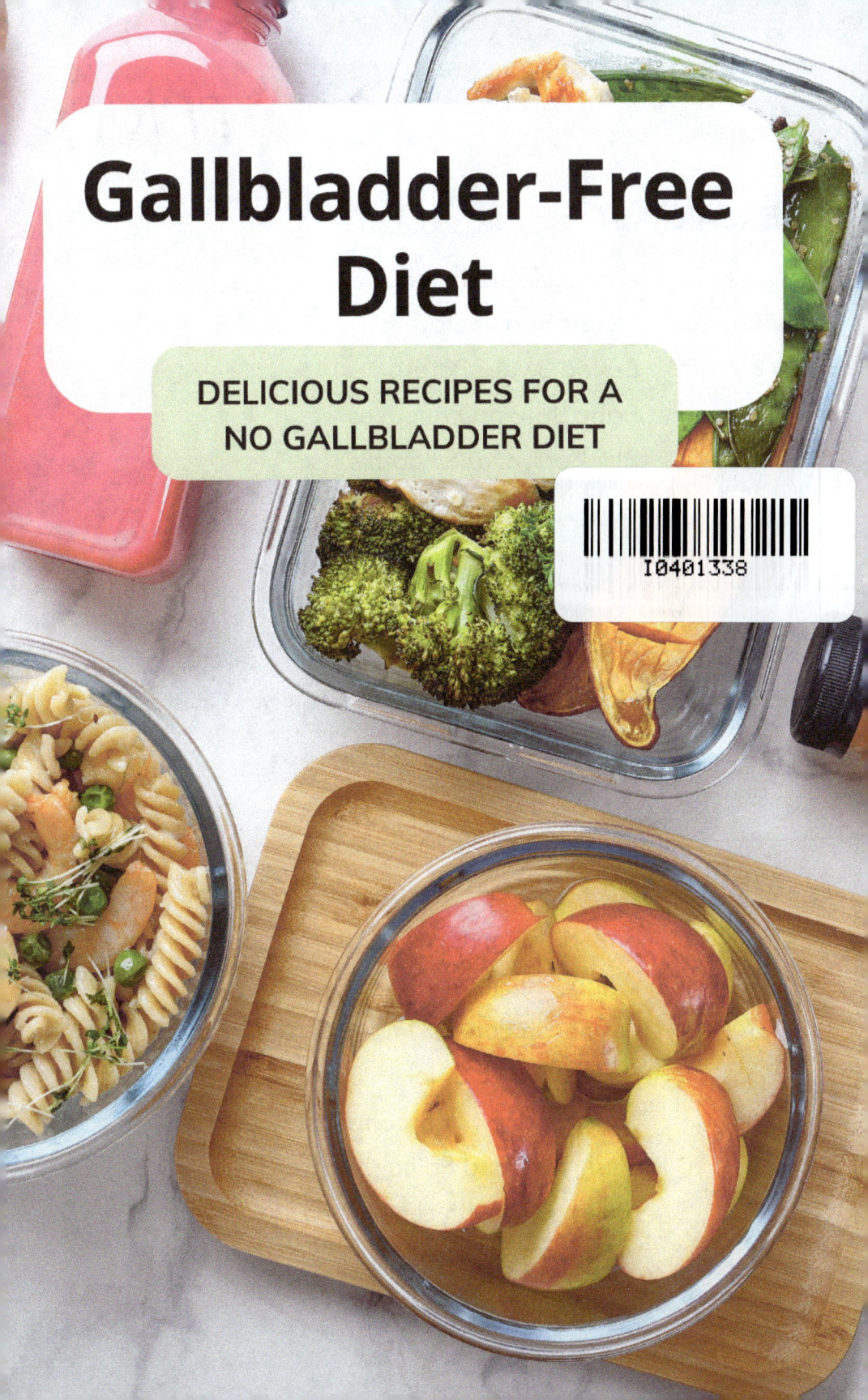

CONTENTS

BREAKFAST

4	Quinoa Breakfast Bowl
6	Mixed Bean Salad
8	Baked Sweet Potato
9	Baby Banana Pancakes
11	Blueberry Oat Smoothie

APPETIZER

14	Spicy Chipotle Grilled Shrimp
17	Black Bean Corn Salsa
19	Slow Roasted Hot Honey Tomato Crostini
21	Smoked Trout Spread
23	Grilled Pineapple

MAIN DISH

27	Baked Italian Chicken and Veggie Foil Packets
29	White Chicken Chili
31	Parmesan Polenta with Roasted Vegetables
33	Honey Garlic Chicken Breast
35	Spinach and Mushroom Soufflé
37	Mushroom and Spinach Frittata
39	Baked Cod with Lemon and Capers
41	Veggie Pizza
43	Grilled Shrimp Kabobs

SIDE DISH

47	Green Bean Casserole
49	Honey Roasted Carrots with Sage
51	Lemony Fava Beans with Garlic and Cilantro
53	Spicy Snow Peas
55	Oven Roasted Beets
56	Lemony Seared Endives
58	Braised Kale And Tomatoes

DESSERT

62	Moist Chocolate Cake
64	Rhubarb Pecan Muffins
66	Lemon Cheesecake
68	Fruit and Nut Bars
70	Easy Red, White, and Blue Parfaits
72	Rice Pudding with Honey Soaked Fruit
74	Strawberry Balsamic Sorbet

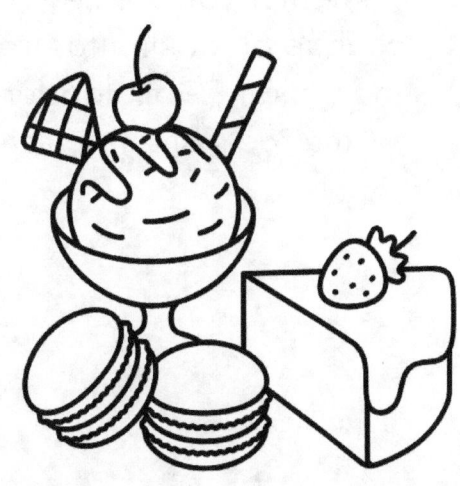

INTRODUCTION

"Gallbladder-Free Gourmet: Delicious Recipes for a No Gallbladder Diet" is your ultimate guide to enjoying flavorful and satisfying meals while maintaining optimal digestive health without a gallbladder. This book offers a carefully curated collection of recipes designed to be gentle on your digestive system, ensuring you can enjoy a diverse range of delicious dishes without discomfort.

This book is perfect for anyone who has undergone gallbladder removal surgery and is seeking guidance on how to adjust their diet without sacrificing flavor or variety. It is also a valuable resource for family members and caregivers who prepare meals for someone without a gallbladder. Whether you are newly adjusting to this dietary change or looking for fresh ideas to enhance your meal plan, "Gallbladder-Free Gourmet" provides the tools and inspiration you need to thrive.

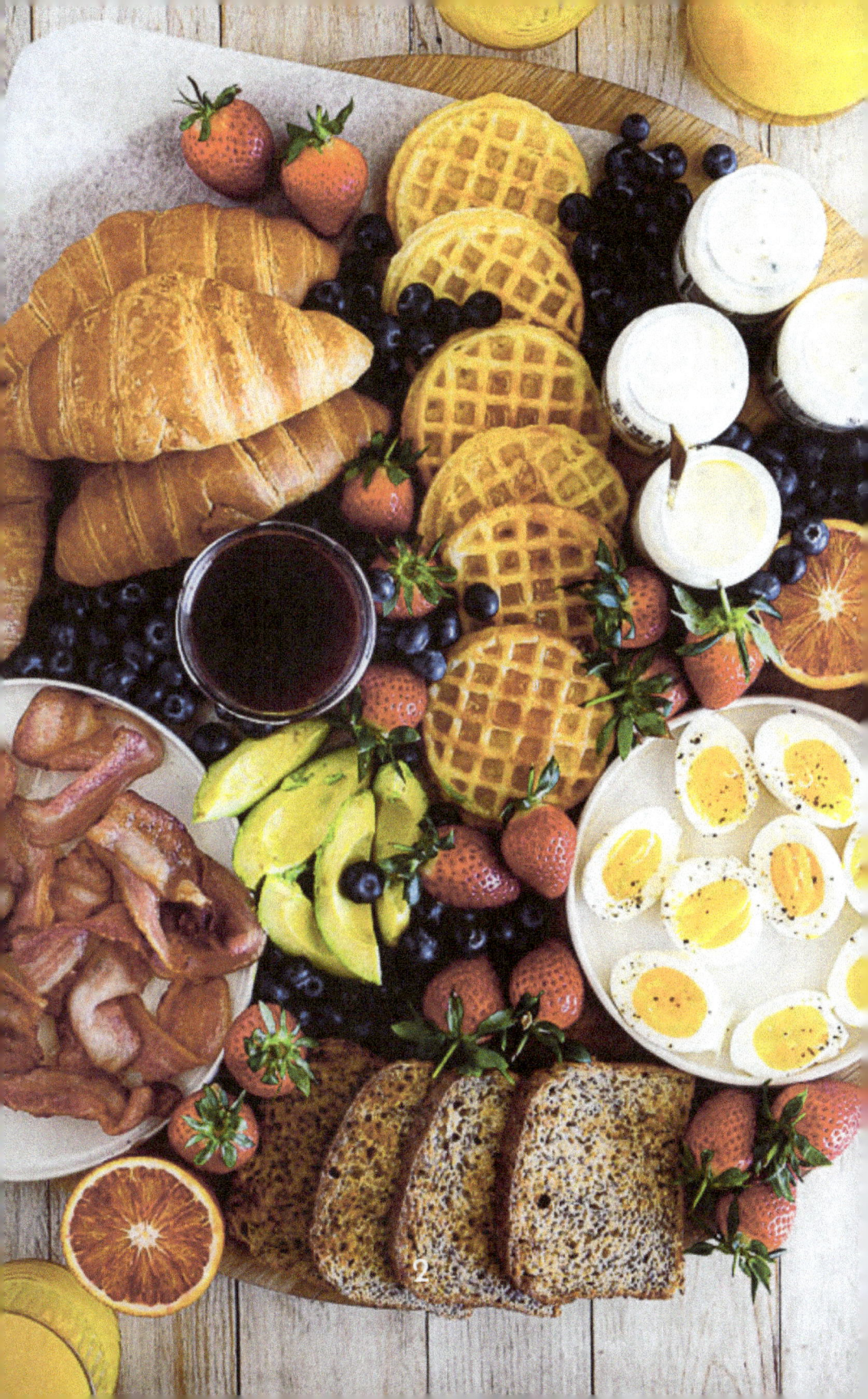

BREAKFAST

Quinoa Breakfast Bowl

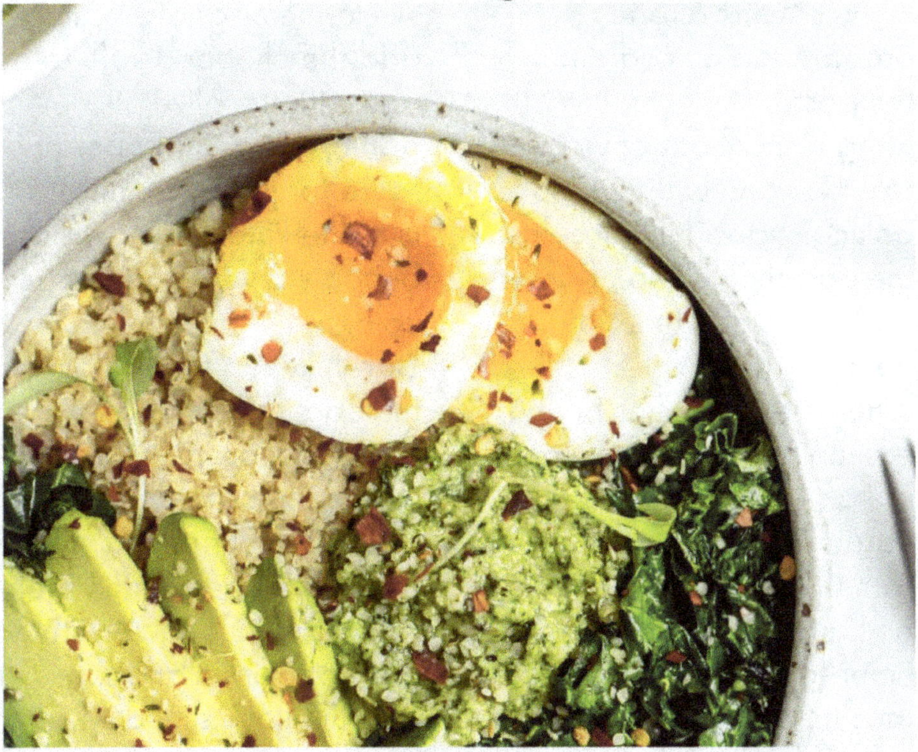

PREP
10 mins

COOK
15 mins

SERVES
2

INGREDIENTS

1 cup cooked quinoa about 1/3 cup dry
2 cups kale chopped finely with the stems removed
1 tablespoon olive oil
1 tablespoon minced garlic
¼ teaspoon salt
¼ teaspoon pepper
½ avocado
4 eggs
½ batch dairy free pesto

INSTRUCTIONS

If you haven't already, prepare the quinoa and the pesto.

Bring a small pot of water to a boil and with 1/2 tsp baking soda. This will help the egg shell come off easily when it's time to peel.

When the water has boiled, reduce the heat to low and use a slotted spoon to carefully add in the eggs. Turn the heat back up to a boil and immediately a timer for 6 1/2 minutes. This amount of time will yield a soft boiled egg, but you can leave the eggs in the boiling water for up to 14 minutes for a hard boiled egg. What I have pictured is 6 1/2 minutes.

Once the time is up, add the eggs into a bowl of ice water. This will immediately stop the cooking process and also make it easier to peel the eggs.

While the eggs are sitting, add the chopped kale to a pan with the olive oil, garlic, salt and pepper and saute for just a few minutes until the kale wilts. It will become a very dark green color.

Carefully tap the bottom of the egg onto a hard surface (a counter works well) to get a crack in the shell. Use your fingers to peel off the rest of the shell. Assemble your bowls with a base of quinoa and top with the kale, sliced avocado, the peeled eggs (sliced in half), pesto and red pepper flakes if desired. Enjoy!

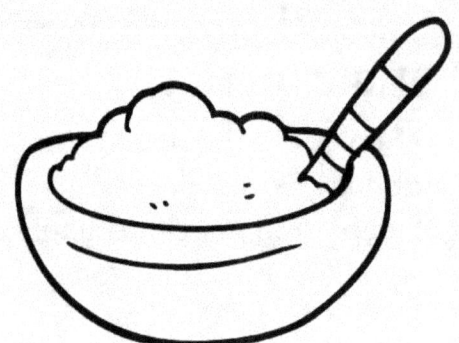

Mixed Bean Salad

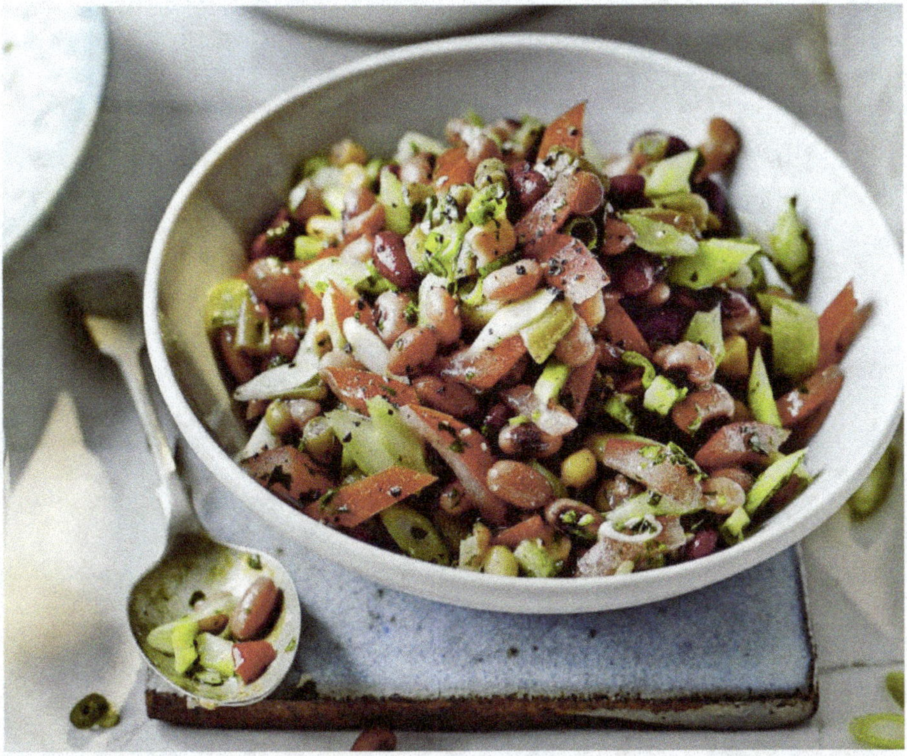

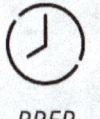

PREP
10 mins

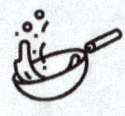

COOK
15 mins

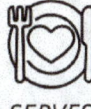

SERVES
2

INGREDIENTS

1 x 400g tin mixed bean salad, drained and rinsed
2 spring onions, finely chopped
2 celery sticks, thinly sliced
1 large tomato, deseeded and finely diced
salt and freshly ground black pepper
3 tbsp olive oil
1 tbsp white wine vinegar
1 tsp sugar
2 tsp Dijon mustard
1 tbsp chopped fresh tarragon

1 tbsp chopped fresh parsley

INSTRUCTIONS

Put all the salad ingredients in a bowl and mix well.

Mix the dressing ingredients in a separate bowl or jug until well combined.

Pour the dressing over the salad, season well with salt and pepper and toss together.

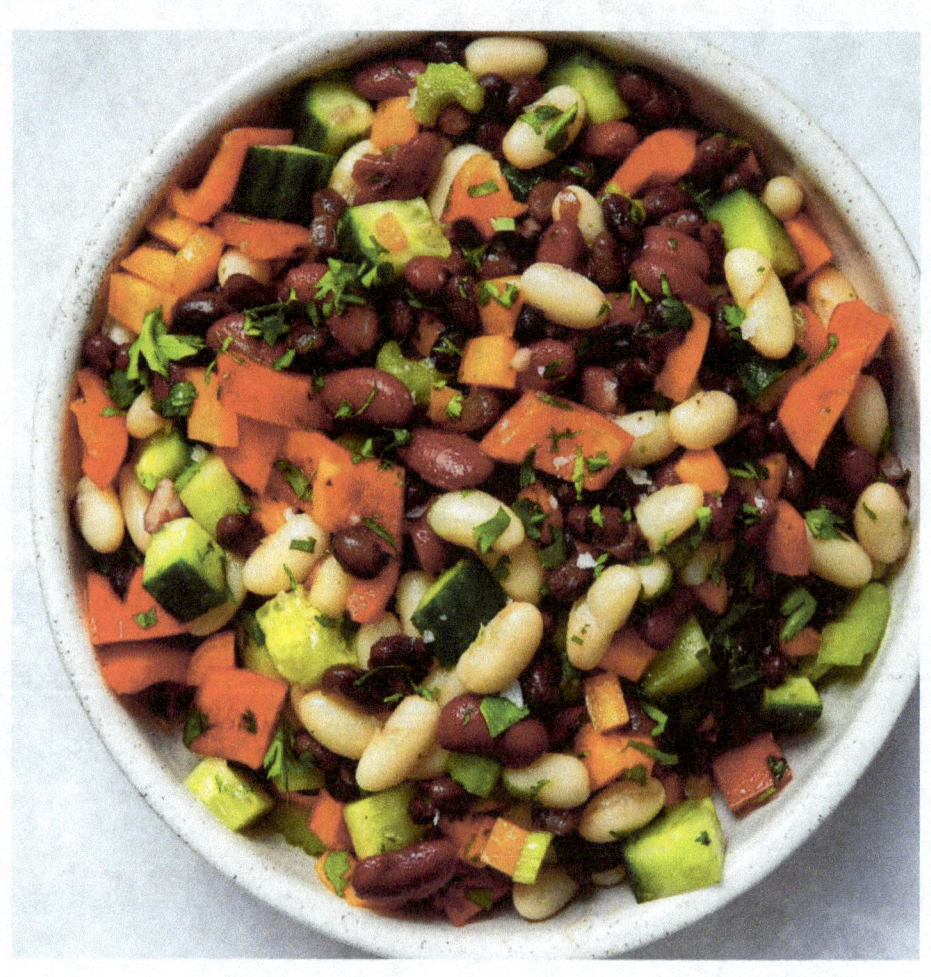

Baked Sweet Potato

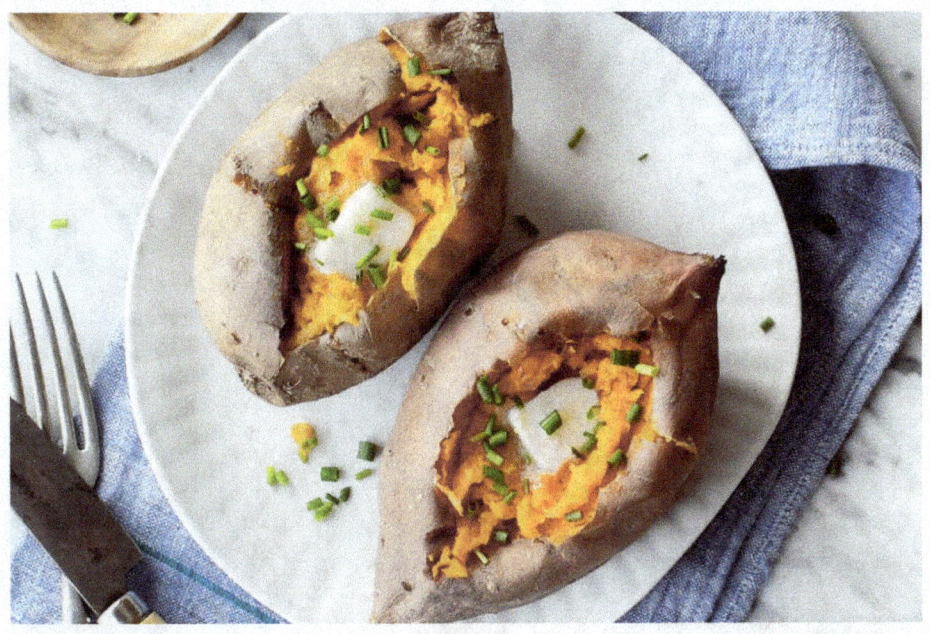

PREP
5 mins

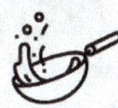

COOK
40 mins

SERVES
4

INGREDIENTS

Sweet Potatoes
Butter or vegan butter,
Sea salt
Chives
Greek yogurt or tzatziki,
Guacamole
Creamy avocado cilantro lime dressing
Any of these stuffing ideas!

INSTRUCTIONS

1. Preheat the oven to 425°F and place a piece of foil on a baking sheet. Use a fork to poke holes into the sweet potatoes, set them on the baking sheet, and roast for 40 to 50 minutes, or until puffed up and soft inside when pierced with a fork.

Baby Banana Pancakes

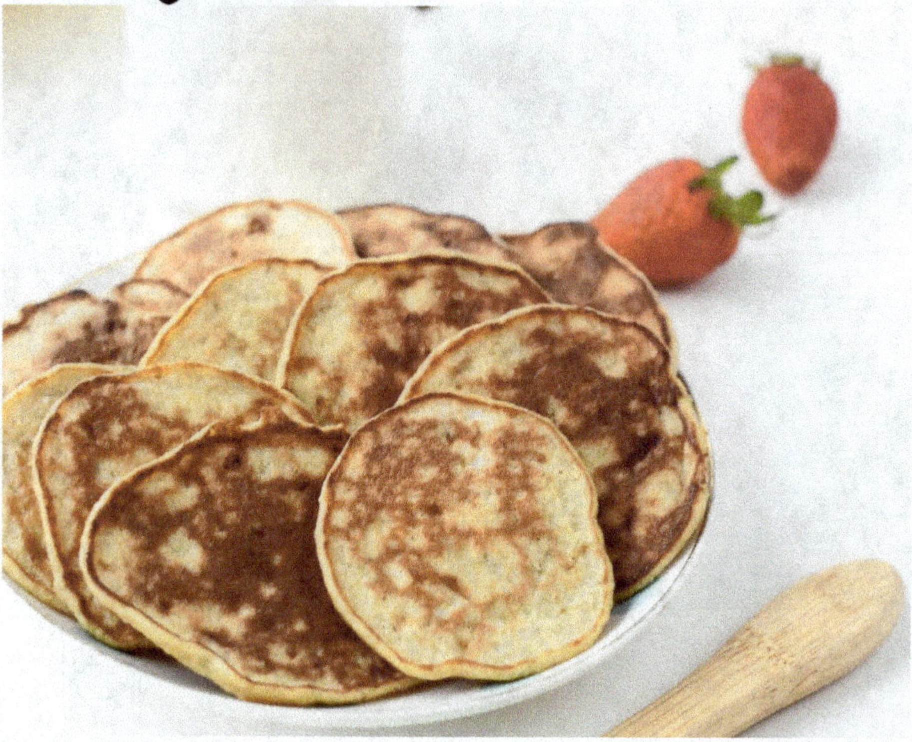

PREP
5 mins

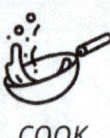
COOK
5 mins

SERVES
8

INGREDIENTS

2 tablespoons Plant-Based Milk - or breast milk
3 tablespoons All-Purpose Flour - or white whole wheat flour
1 small Banana - riped, peeled

INSTRUCTIONS

Peel and mash the ripe banana on a plate until smooth. It's OK if bits of banana show.

Stir the milk and mashed banana, then stir in the flour.

Whisk everything together and set the pancake batter aside for 5 minutes while the pancake griddle warms up.

Lightly grease the pancake griddle with coconut oil.

Pour 1 tablespoon of batter per pancake and cook for 1-2 minutes or until the sides start to dry out.

Flip the pancakes and cook them for an extra 30-60 seconds.

Let the pancakes cool on a cooling rack for 10 minutes, then serve them plain or with the baby jam recipe.

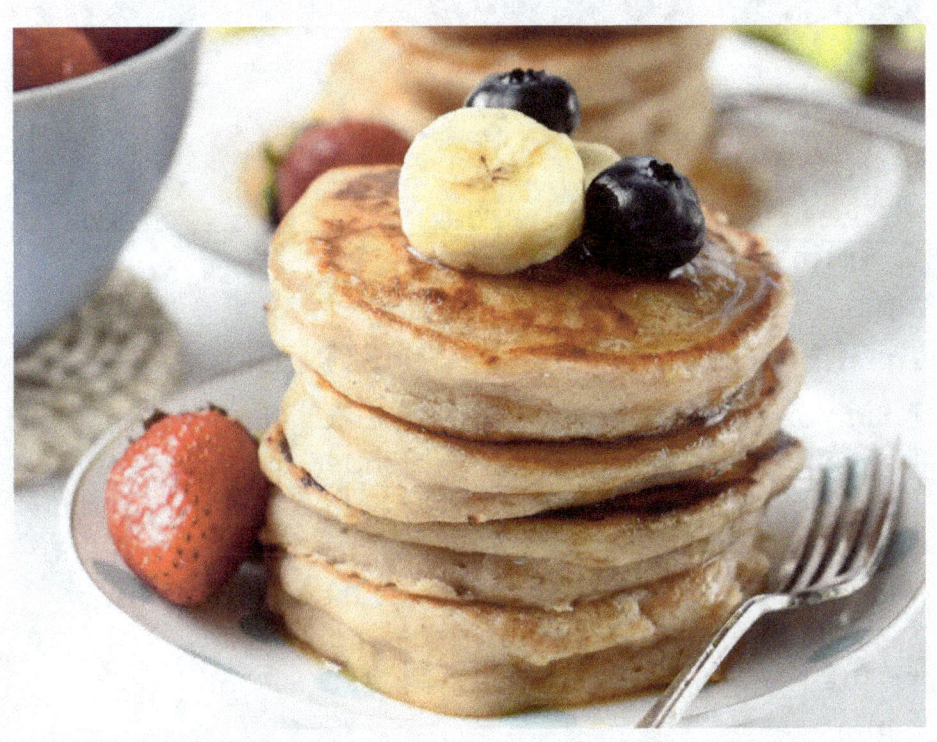

Blueberry Oat Smoothie

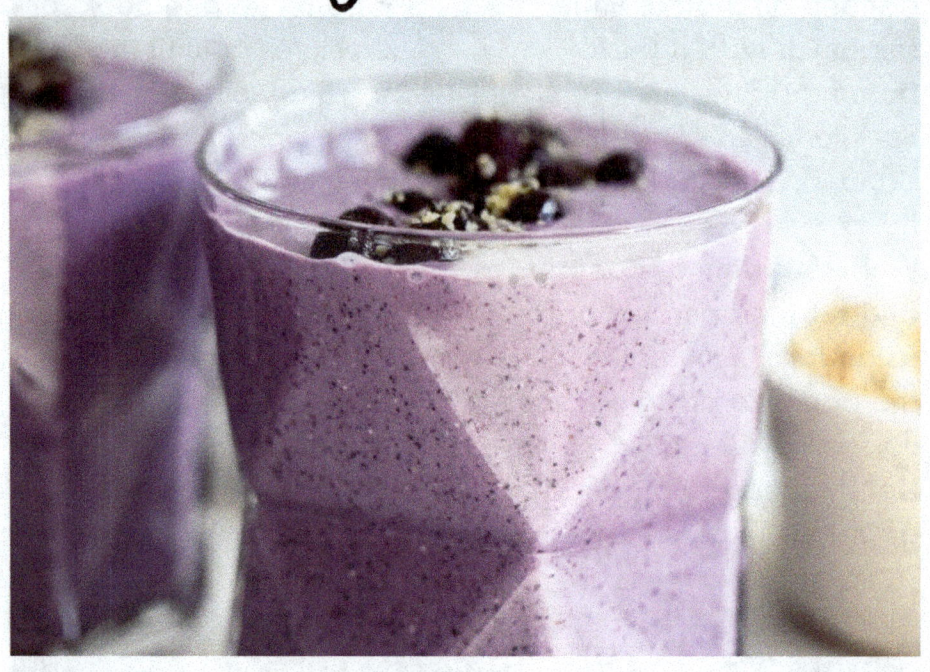

PREP
5 mins

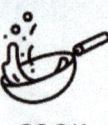
COOK
5 mins

SERVES
2

INGREDIENTS

1 cup frozen blueberries
1 banana
1 cup plain, non-dairy milk
1/2 cup plain or vanilla vegan yogurt
1/3 cup old fashioned oats
1 tablespoon almond butter
1 teaspoon vanilla extract

INSTRUCTIONS

Place all ingredients in a blender and puree until smooth. (You can blend the oats until finely ground first and then add the rest of the ingredients.)

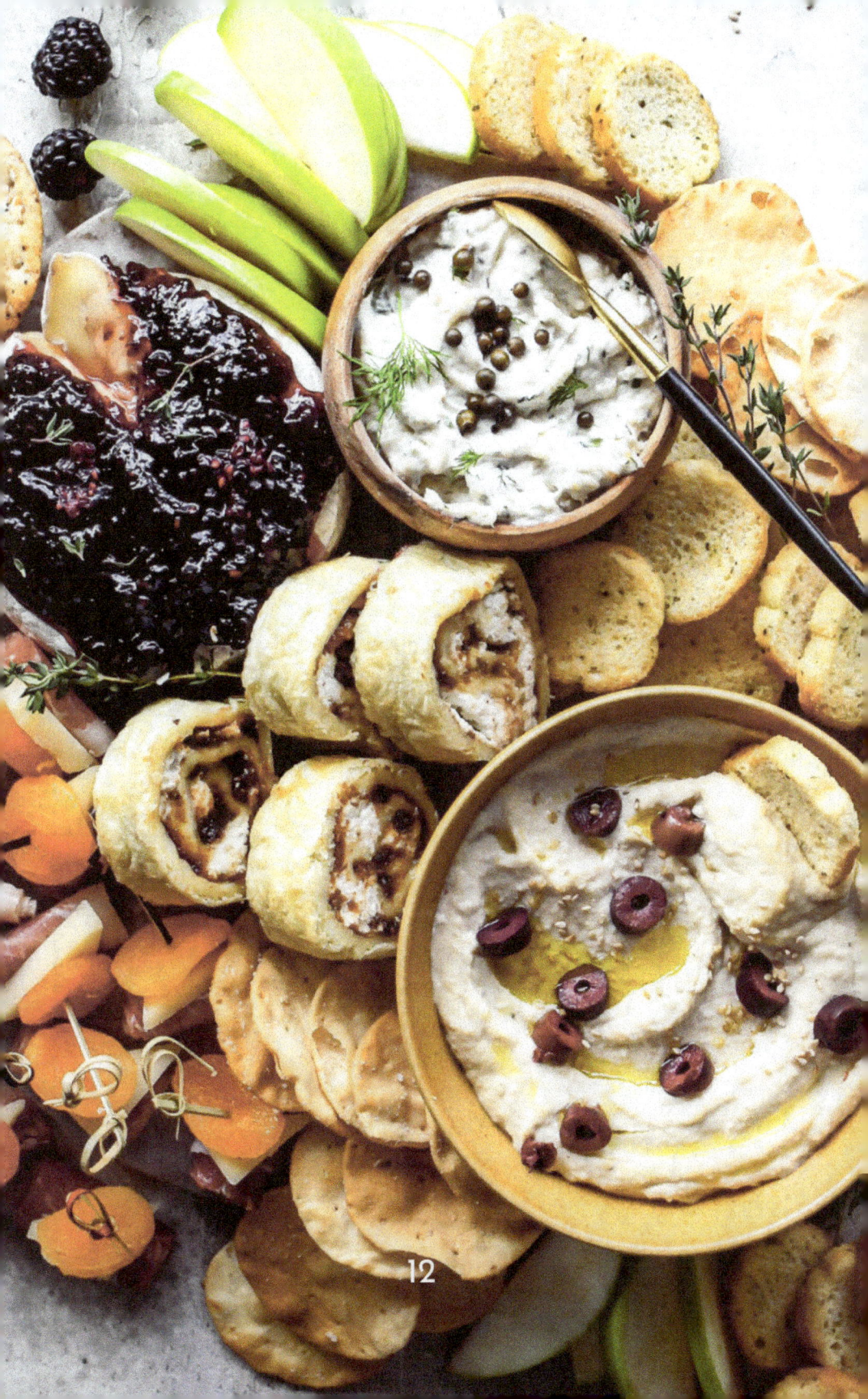

APPETIZER

Spicy Chipotle Grilled Shrimp

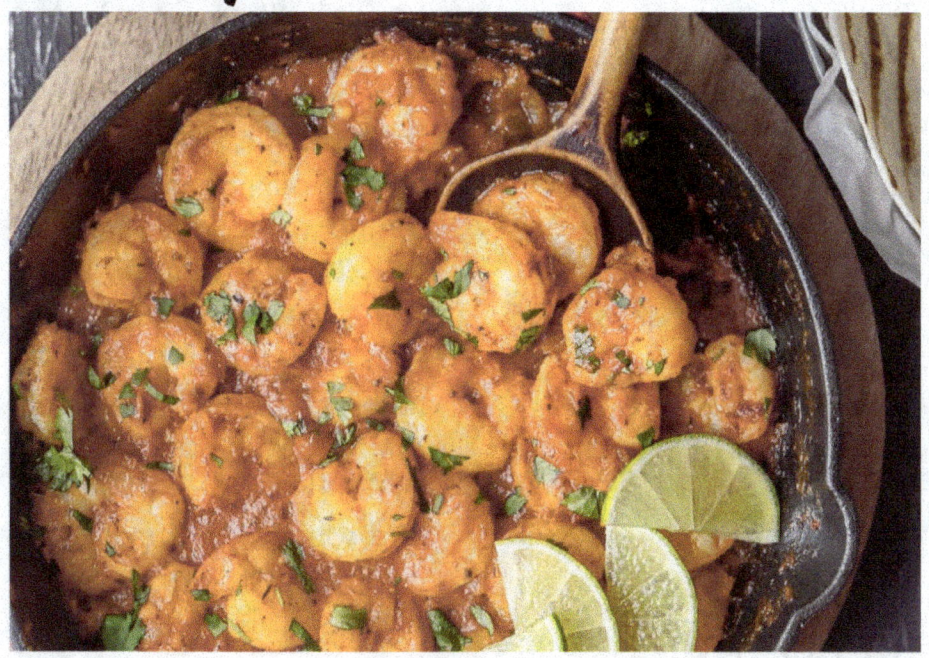

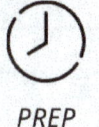

PREP
5 mins

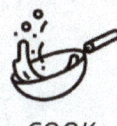

COOK
20 mins

SERVES
4

INGREDIENTS

1 14.5 oz can Fire-Roasted Tomatoes
2-4 chipotle chilies in adobo sauce plus the sauce clinging to them
Kosher salt
Freshly ground black pepper
¼ cup olive oil
1½ lb. extra-large raw shrimp; peeled deveined, tails removed and patted dry

¼ cup fresh lime juice divided
½ medium sweet yellow onion diced
4 garlic cloves peeled and minced
½ teaspoon dried oregano
¼ cup dry white wine
½ cup chopped cilantro plus extra for garnish
For serving:
8 6-inch corn tortillas, warmed
avocado slices
sour cream or Mexican crema
lime wedges

INSTRUCTIONS

Preheat oven to 200 degrees F. Stack the tortillas, wrap them in foil then place in the oven to warm while preparing the shrimp.

In a food processor, place the tomatoes, chilies (plus sauce clinging from them) and ¾ teaspoon kosher salt. Pulse 1 minute or until almost smooth.

In a 12-inch nonstick skillet, heat 2 tablespoons oil over medium-high heat just until it begins to smoke. Add half the shrimp and cook 45 seconds, turning often. Transfer the cooked shrimp to a bowl and repeat with the remaining shrimp. Place the remaining cooked shrimp in the bowl and mix with 2 tablespoons of the lime juice.

Turn the heat to medium-high and add the remaining 2 tablespoons oil to the skillet. Add the onion and sauté for 3-4 minutes; add garlic and oregano and cook just until it begins to brown, about 1 minute. Stir in the wine and the leftover shrimp juice from the bowl. Cook until liquid is nearly evaporated. Turn heat to low and add half of the prepared chipotle sauce. Simmer, stirring, until the mixture thickens enough to coat the back of a spoon, approximately 10-12 minutes.

Remove the skillet from the heat and add the shrimp; stir gently. Cover and let sit until the shrimp are opaque and cooked through, 2-4 minutes. Add the cilantro and remaining lime juice, stir.

Taste, then season with salt and pepper, if needed. Serve with warmed tortillas, slices of avocado, sour cream or Mexican crema and lime wedges.
Enjoy!

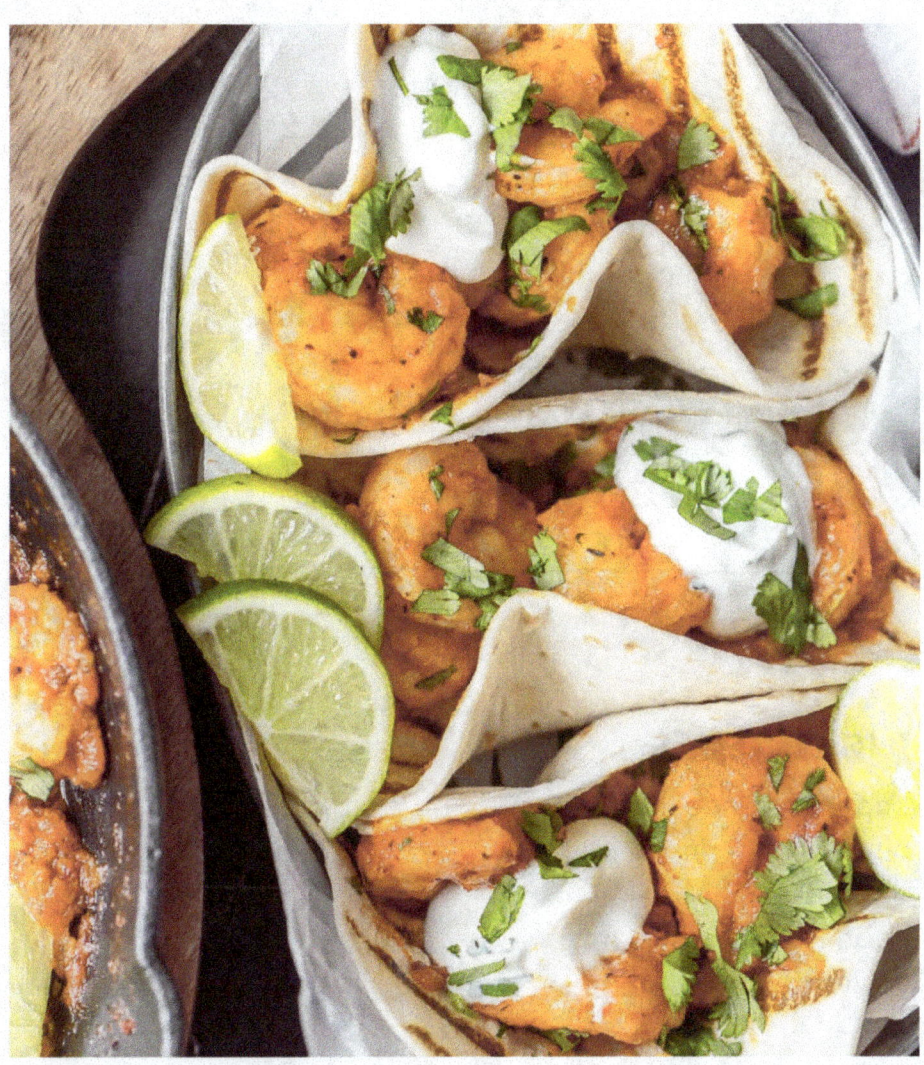

Black Bean Corn Salsa

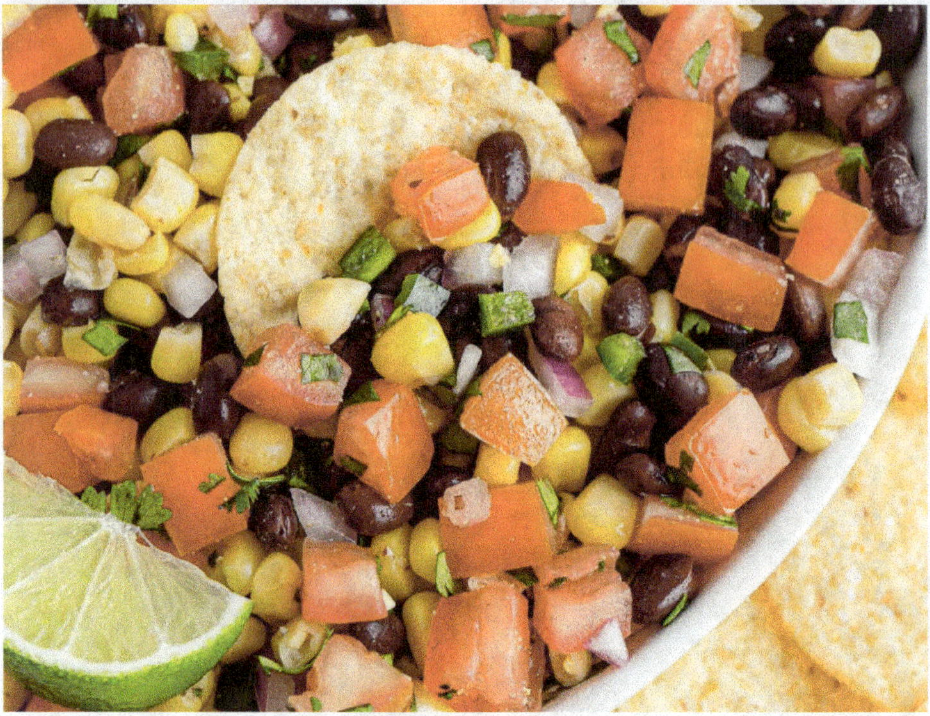

PREP
20 mins

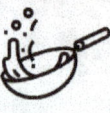
COOK
2 mins

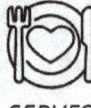
SERVES
8

INGREDIENTS

1 can (15 ounces) black or pinto beans, rinsed and drained

1 can (15 ounces) corn, drained

1 ½ cups finely chopped roma tomatoes, seeds removed (about 3 tomatoes)

¼ cup finely diced red onion, finely diced (about ¼ onion)

1 jalapeño pepper, seeds and ribs removed, finely diced
¼ cup minced cilantro (leaves and small stems)
2 tablespoons fresh lime juice (from 1 lime)
½ teaspoon ground cumin
½ teaspoon kosher salt
⅛ teaspoon coarse ground black pepper

INSTRUCTIONS

In medium sized bowl, combine all ingredients. Refrigerate until ready to serve.

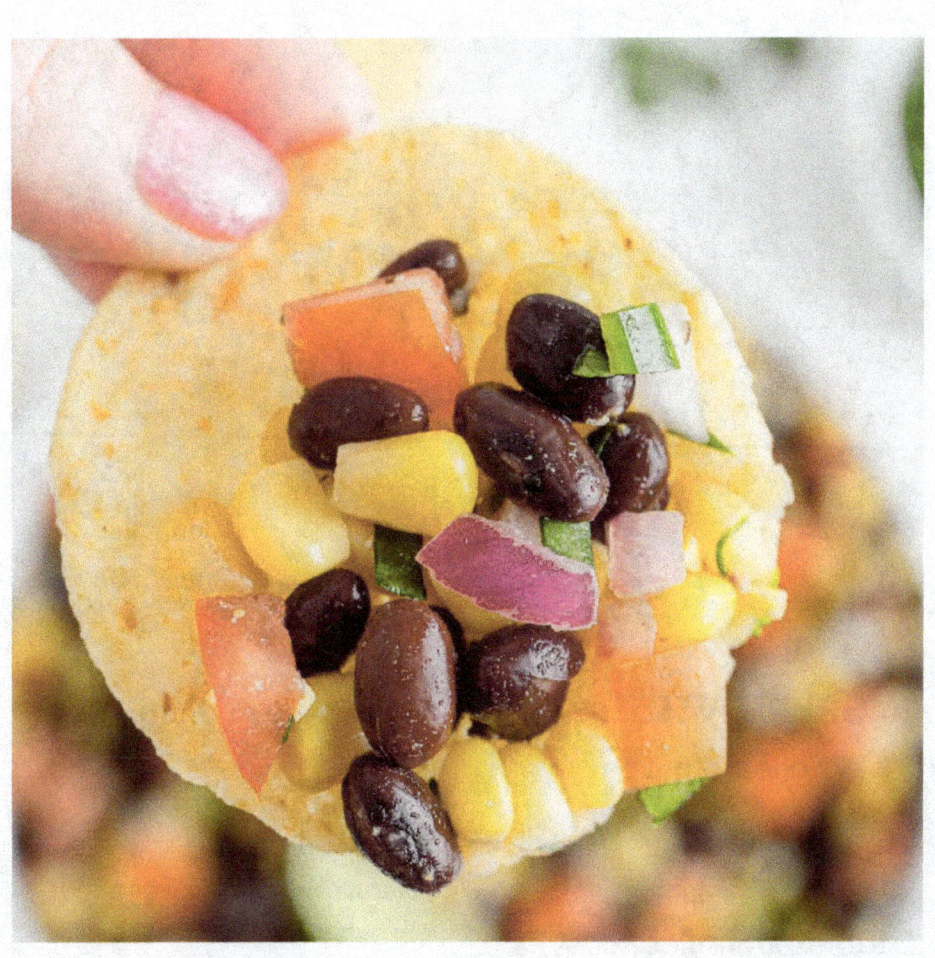

Slow Roasted Hot Honey Tomato Crostini

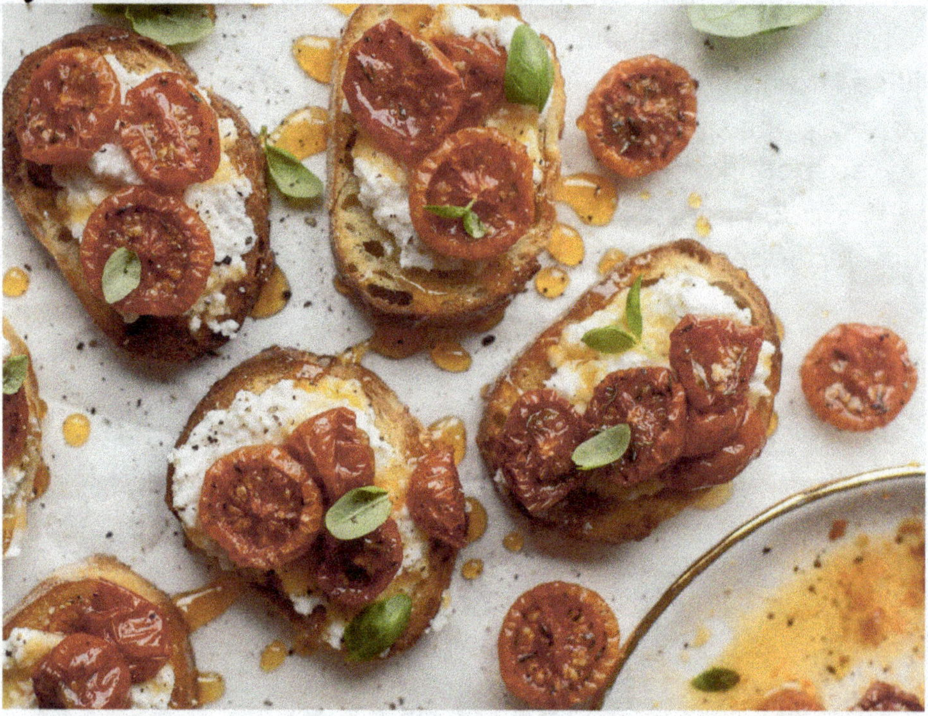

PREP
2 hours

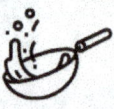
COOK
15 mins

SERVES
8

INGREDIENTS

2 pints cherry/grape tomatoes halved
1 tablespoon olive oil, plus more for drizzling
2 tablespoons hot honey, plus extra for drizzling
½ teaspoon dried thyme
kosher salt and pepper
1 large baguette, sliced into rounds
1 cup ricotta cheese
fresh basil, for topping

INSTRUCTIONS

Preheat the oven to 300 degrees F. Line a baking sheet with parchment paper.
Place the cherry tomatoes on the sheet and drizzle with olive oil. Drizzle with the hot honey. Sprinkle with a big pinch of salt and pepper. Sprinkle with the thyme. Roast for 1.5 to 2 hours, tossing every 30 minutes, until the tomatoes are super caramely and shriveled and sweet. Remove the tomatoes and let them cool. While cooling, increase the oven temperature to 350 degrees F. Place the baguette slices on a baking sheet. Drizzle with olive oil. Roast for 8 to 10 minutes, until golden.

To serve, spread the crostini with a dollop of ricotta cheese. Drizzle with hot honey. Top with the slow roasted tomatoes. Add a few basil leaves. Serve!

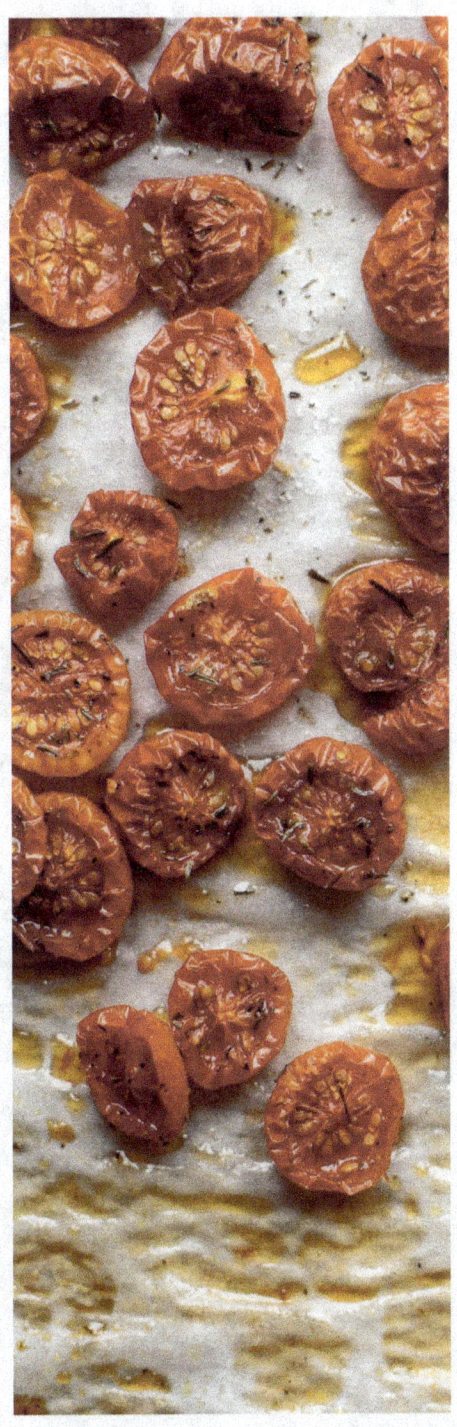

Smoked Trout Spread

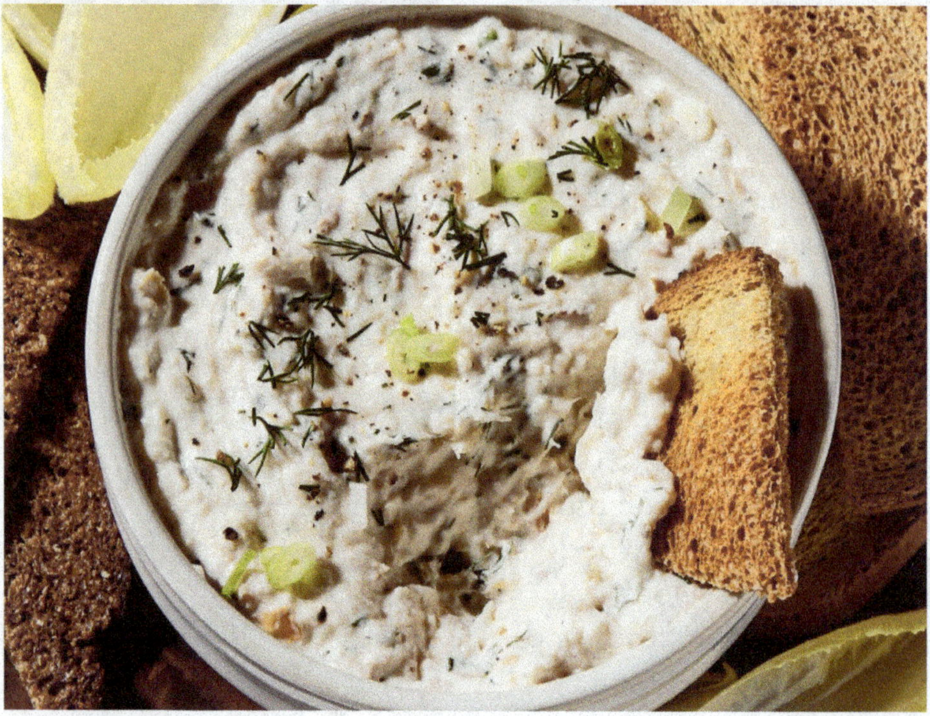

PREP
15 mins

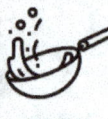
COOK
3 hours

SERVES
8-10

INGREDIENTS

8 oz. smoked trout, bones and skin removed
4 oz. cream cheese, room temperature
1/4 c. sour cream
1/4 c. mixed chopped scallions, dill, and/or chives, plus more for serving
1 Tbsp. fresh lemon juice
1 Tbsp. prepared horseradish

1/2 tsp. (or more) fish sauce (optional)
1/4 tsp. (or more) kosher salt
1/4 tsp. (or more) freshly ground black pepper
Toasted bread, crackers, and/or crudités, for serving

INSTRUCTIONS

1. Using 2 forks, flake trout into small, bite-sized pieces. In a large bowl, mix trout, cream cheese, and sour cream with a spatula until well combined. Fold in scallions and herbs, lemon juice, horseradish, fish sauce (if using), salt, and pepper. Cover and refrigerate at least 3 hours or up to overnight.

2. When ready to serve, taste dip and adjust seasonings. Transfer to a serving dish and top with scallions and herbs. Serve with bread alongside.

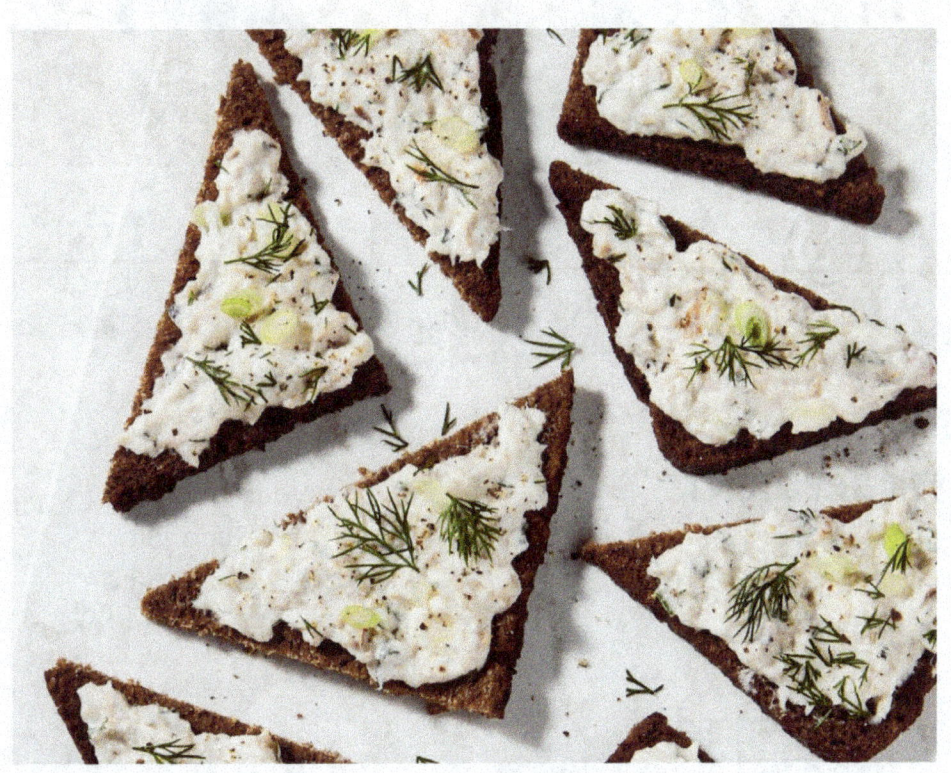

Grilled Pineapple

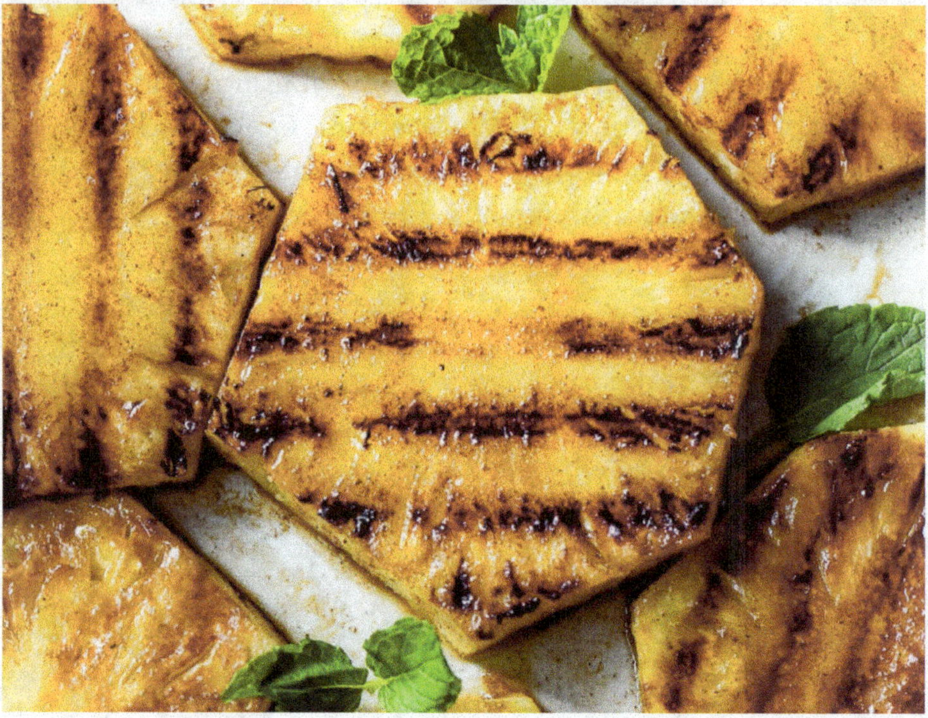

PREP
5 mins

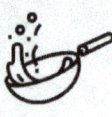
COOK
10 mins

SERVES
4

INGREDIENTS

8 pineapple slices, 1/2 inch thick (from 1 pineapple)

For the marinade:
2 tbsp dark honey

1 tsp olive oil
1 tbsp fresh lime juice
1 tsp ground cinnamon
ice cream, optional for topping

INSTRUCTIONS

In a small bowl, combine the honey, olive oil, lime juice, and cinnamon and whisk to blend. Set aside. Heat the grill or a grill pan over medium-high heat. When hot, lightly coat the grates with oil spray.
Lightly brush the pineapple with the marinade.
Grill turning once and basting once or twice with the remaining marinade, until tender and golden, about 3-4 minutes on each side.
Serve warm.

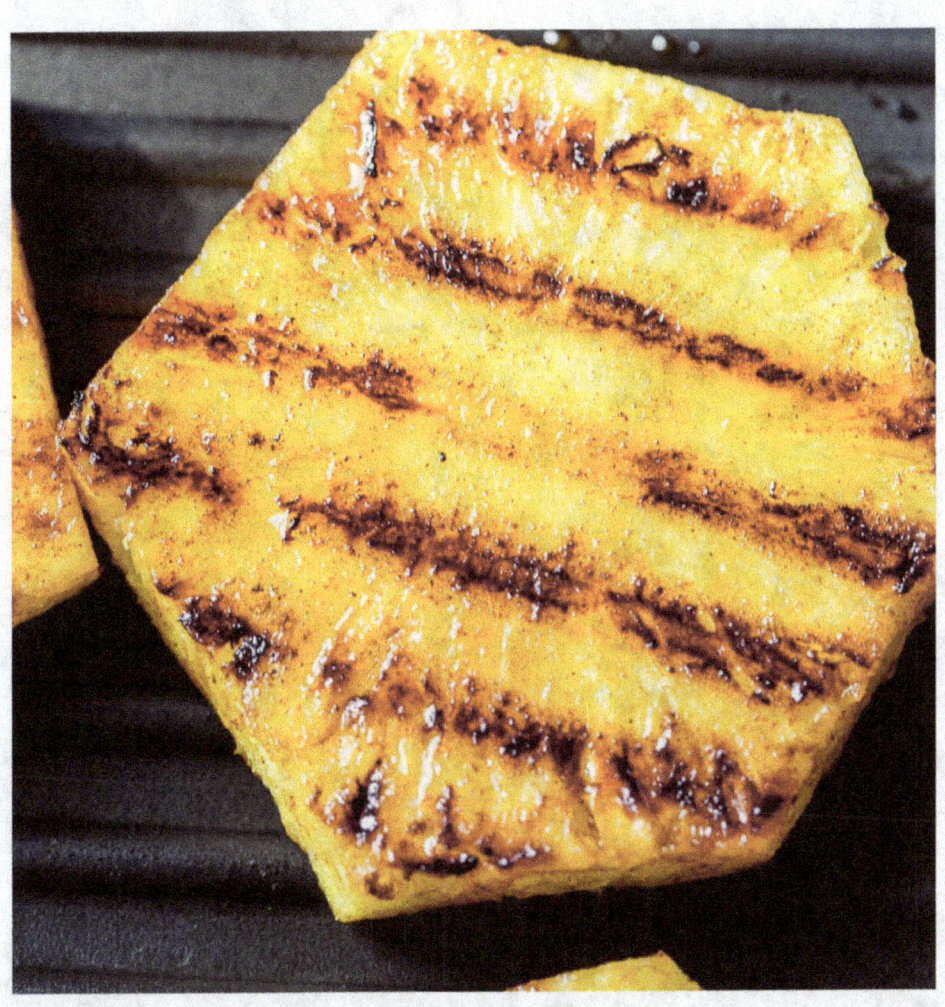

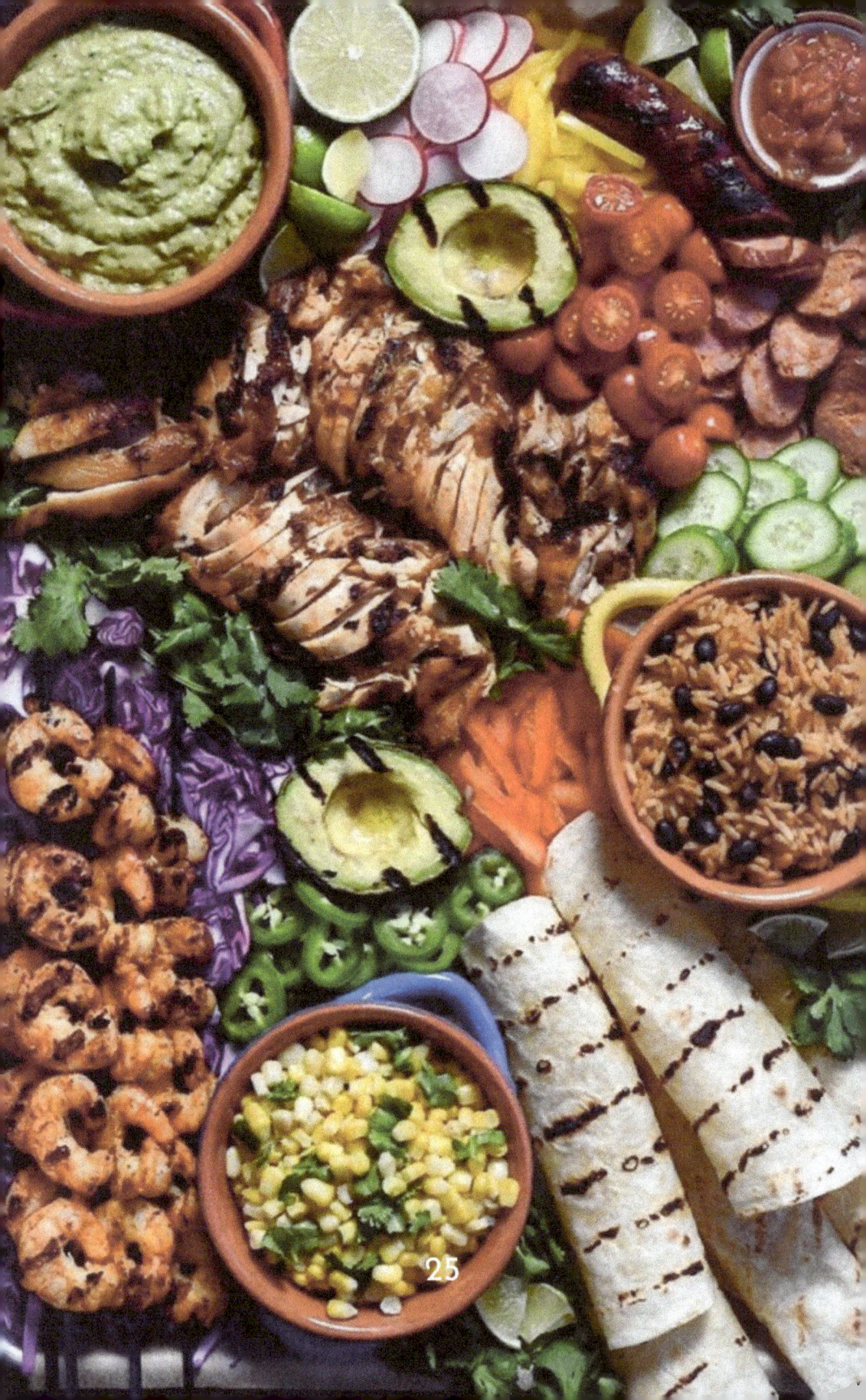

MAIN DISH

Baked Italian Chicken and Veggie Foil Packets

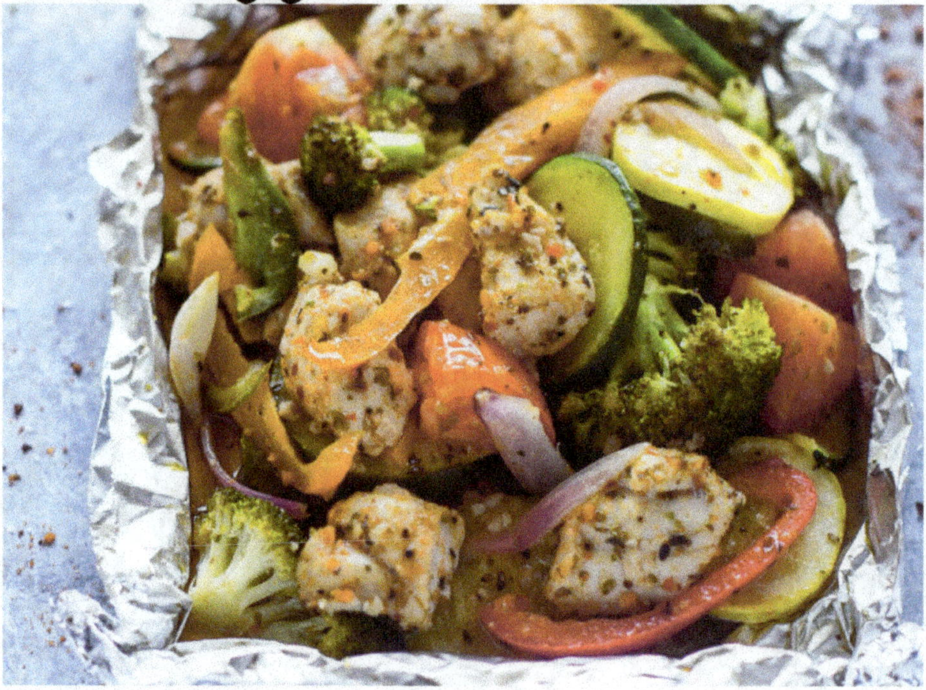

PREP
10 mins

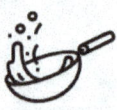
COOK
20 mins

SERVES
2

INGREDIENTS

2 small, or 1 large chicken breasts cut into 1 inch cubes
1 cup broccoli florets
1 cup bell peppers, sliced or chopped (colors of choice)
1 small zucchini, sliced
1/2 cup tomatoes sliced into large chunks

1/2 cup onion, sliced or chopped
1 tablespoon olive oil
1 tablespoon italian seasoning *, see note
1 teaspoon garlic powder or fresh minced garlic
1 teaspoon paprika, optional
salt and pepper to taste

INSTRUCTIONS

Pre-heat oven to 400F.

In a large bowl combine or ziplock bag, combine all the ingredients and mix until fully combined.

Cut and lay out 2 12x12 inch (app.) squares of aluminum foil on a sheet pan. Place half the mixture on each foil and gently fold the foil around ingredients to form a tight seal.

Bake for 20 minutes or until chicken is cooked through. Serve with a side of rice or noodles.

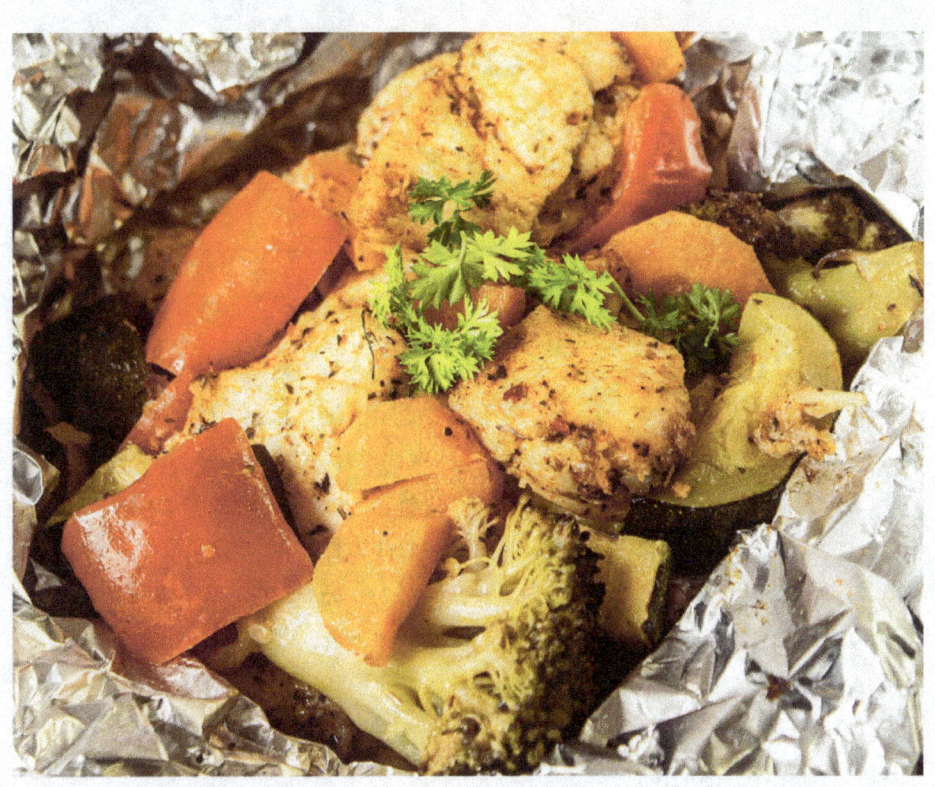

White Chicken Chili

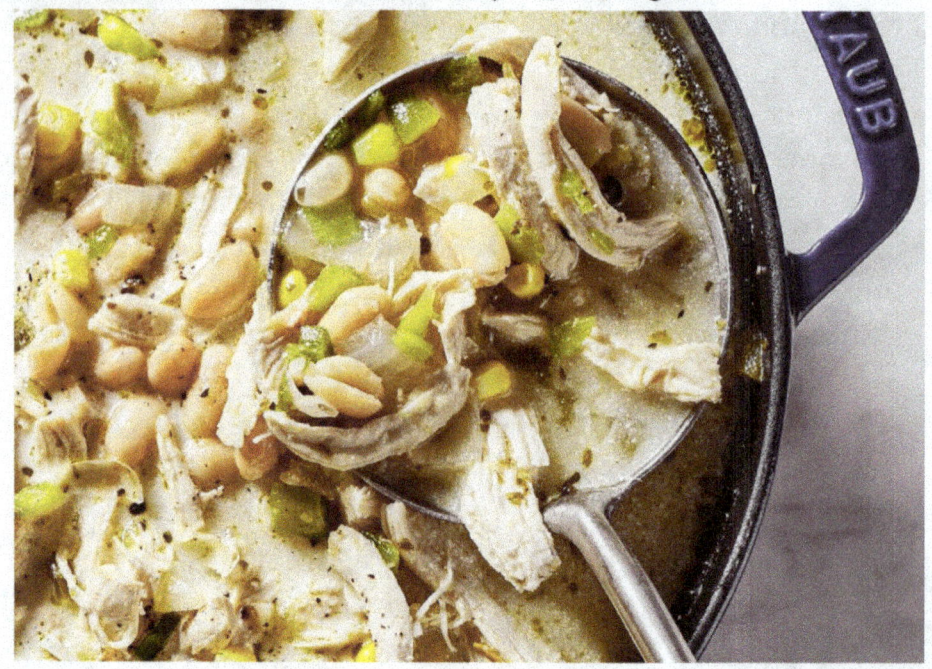

PREP
25 mins

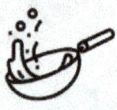
COOK
20 mins

SERVES
6

INGREDIENTS

1 Tbsp. neutral oil
1 medium yellow onion, chopped
1 jalapeño, seeded, finely chopped
2 cloves garlic, finely chopped
1 tsp. dried oregano
1 tsp. ground cumin
3 boneless, skinless chicken breasts, cut into thirds
5 c. low-sodium chicken broth
2 (4.5-oz.) cans green chiles
Kosher salt
Freshly ground black pepper

2 (15-oz.) cans white beans, drained, rinsed
1 1/2 c. frozen corn
1/2 c. sour cream
1 avocado, thinly sliced, for serving
1/4 c. chopped fresh cilantro, for serving
1/4 c. crushed tortilla chips, for serving
1/4 c. shredded Monterey Jack, for serving

INSTRUCTIONS

In a large pot over medium heat, heat oil. Add onion and jalapeño and cook, stirring, until softened, about 8 minutes. Add garlic, oregano, and cumin and cook, stirring, until fragrant, about 1 minute. Add chicken, broth, and chiles; season with salt and pepper. Bring to a boil, then reduce heat and simmer, uncovered, until chicken is tender and cooked through, 10 to 12 minutes. Transfer chicken to a plate and shred with 2 forks. Add beans to pot and bring to a simmer. Cook, smashing about one-quarter of beans with a wooden spoon, until slightly thickened, about 10 minutes. Add corn and shredded chicken and cook, stirring, until heated through, about 1 minute more. Remove from heat and stir in sour cream. Ladle chili into bowls. Top with avocado, cilantro, chips, and cheese.

Parmesan Polenta with Roasted Vegetables

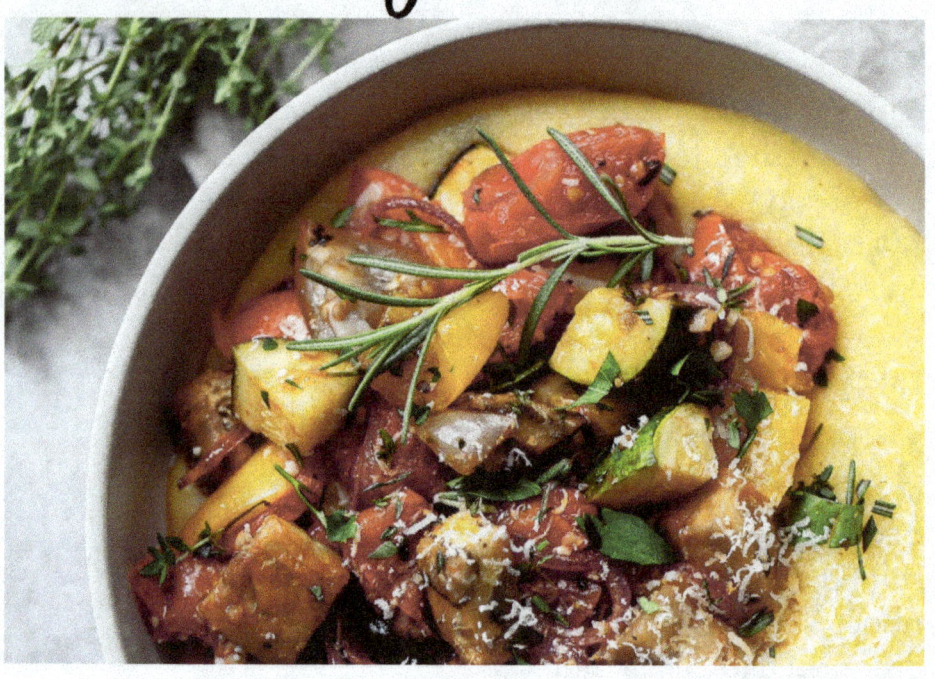

PREP
10 mins

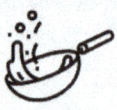
COOK
30 mins

SERVES
4

INGREDIENTS

2 bell peppers in assorted colors, chopped into 1/2-inch pieces

1 small eggplant, cut into 1-inch cubes (1-1/2 cups)

1 pint grape or cherry tomatoes, halved

3 small or 2 medium-sized zucchini, cut into 1-inch chunks

½ red onion, thinly sliced

2 tablespoons (30 ml) extra-virgin olive oil
½ teaspoon kosher salt
2 garlic cloves, finely chopped
½ teaspoon crushed red chili flakes
2 teaspoons chopped fresh thyme or rosemary
tablespoon balsamic vinegar
1 cup (160 g) coarse cornmeal
1-2 teaspoons salt
½ cup freshly grated Parmesan cheese
4 tablespoons (60 g) butter

INSTRUCTIONS

Combine the peppers, eggplant, tomatoes, zucchini, onion, olive oil and the salt on a large rimmed baking sheet. Roast until beginning to soften and turn brown, 20-25 minutes. Remove the pan from the oven and stir in the garlic, chili, thyme and balsamic vinegar.

Bring 4 cups of water to a boil in a heavy-duty sauce pan or small Dutch oven. Stir in 1 teaspoon salt. Gradually sprinkle the polenta into the pan while whisking at the same time. Turn the heat to a very low simmer, cover and continue to cook the polenta for 25-30 minutes, until it's thick, fluffy and begins to pull away from the sides of the pan. Stir occasionally so it doesn't stick to the bottom of the pan. When it's done remove from the heat and stir in the cheese, butter and additional salt to taste, if needed.

Spoon the warm polenta into bowls and put some of the roasted vegetables and the pan juice over each serving. Sprinkle with additional cheese, if you like.

Honey Garlic Chicken Breast

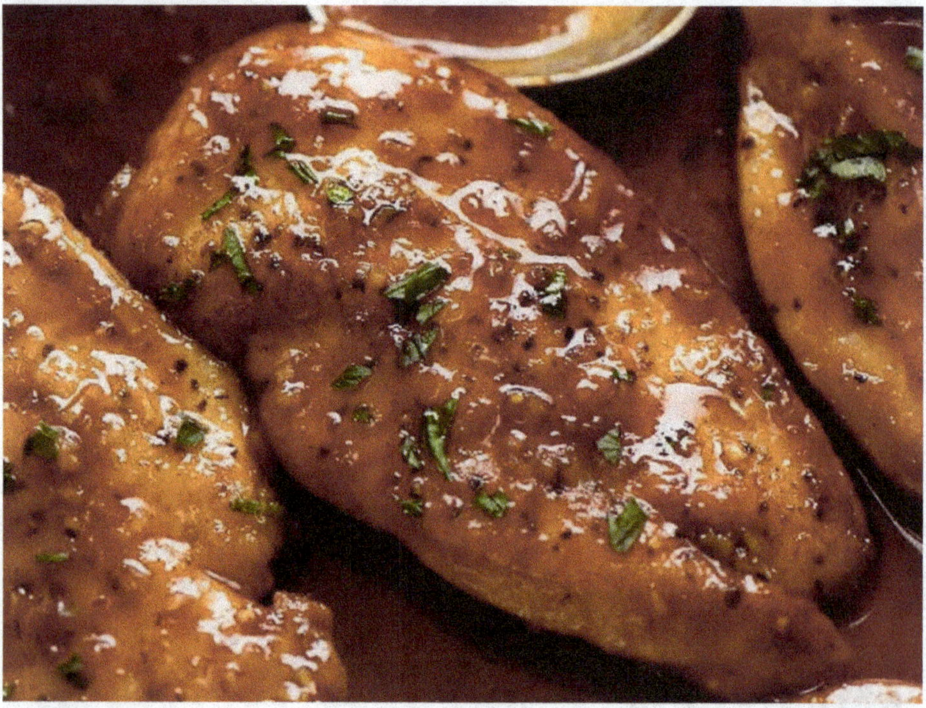

PREP
4 mins

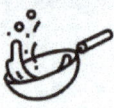
COOK
8 mins

SERVES
4

INGREDIENTS

500g / 1 lb chicken breast , boneless and skinless (2 pieces)
Salt and pepper
1/4 cup flour (Note 1)

3 1/2 tbsp (50g) unsalted butter (or 2 1/2 tbsp olive oil)
2 garlic cloves , minced
1 1/2 tbsp apple cider vinegar (or white or other clear vinegar)

1 tbsp soy sauce , light or all purpose
1/3 cup honey (or maple syrup)

INSTRUCTIONS

Cut the breasts in half horizontally to create 4 steaks in total. Sprinkle each side with salt and pepper.
Place flour in a shallow dish. Coat chicken in flour and shake off excess.
Melt most of the butter in a large skillet over high heat – hold back about 1 tsp for later.
Place chicken in skillet and cook for 2 – 3 minutes until golden. Turn and cook the other side for 1 minute.
Turn heat down slightly to medium high.
Make a bit of room in the pan and add garlic and top with remaining dab of butter. Stir garlic briefly once butter melts.
Add vinegar, soy sauce and honey. Stir / shake pan to combine. Bring sauce to simmer, then simmer for 1 minute or until slightly thickened.
Turn chicken to coat in sauce. If the sauce gets too thick, add a touch of water and stir.
Remove from stove immediately. Place chicken on plates and drizzle over remaining sauce.

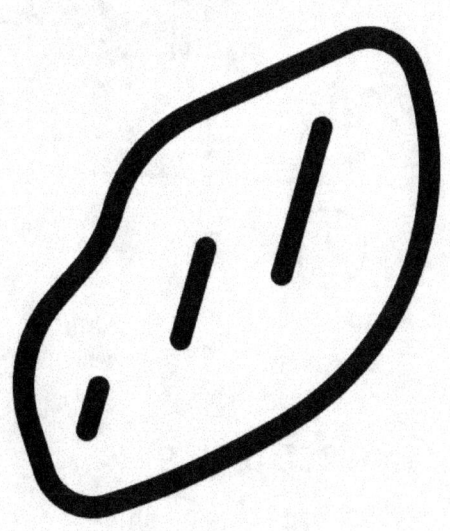

Spinach and Mushroom Soufflé

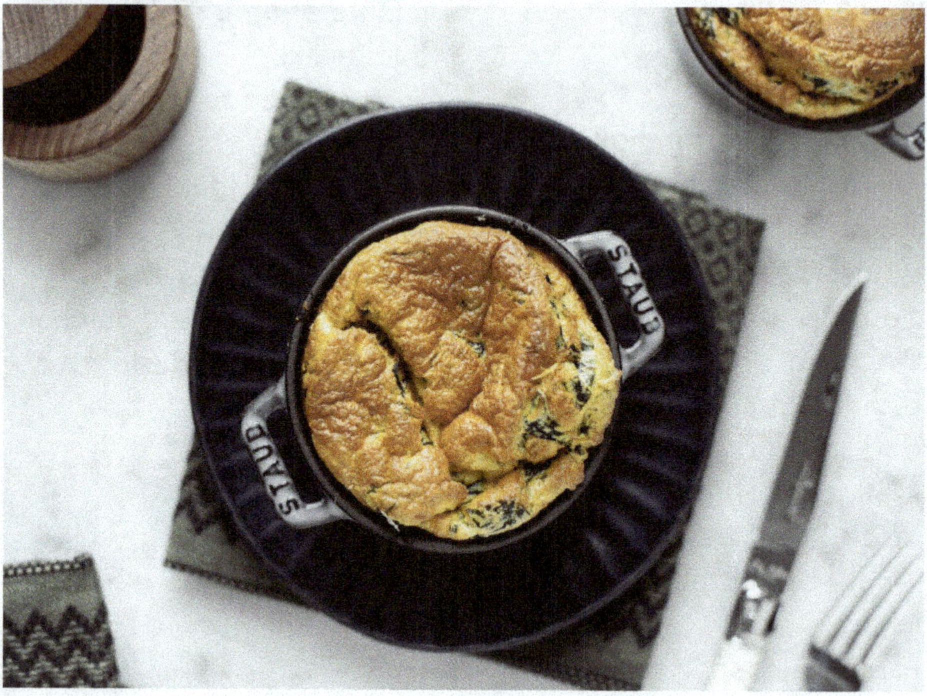

PREP
15 mins

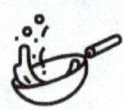
COOK
15 mins

SERVES
4

INGREDIENTS

3 tablespoons freshly grated parmesan cheese
16 ounces fresh spinach, stemmed & chopped
1 cup white or cremini mushrooms, thinly sliced
3 tablespoons unsalted butter
3 tablespoons all purpose flour
1 clove of garlic, grated
1 cup whole milk, hot

Salt & pepper, to taste
1 pinch nutmeg, optional
4 large eggs, separated
1/2 cup grated swiss cheese
1 pinch cream of tartar

INSTRUCTIONS

1. Preheat oven to 400(f) degrees. Butter the inside of 4 large or 6 small ramekins. Sprinkle evenly with parmesan.
2. In a saucepan pan over low heat add the spinach & mushrooms. Cook until spinach is wilted & liquid has evaporated. Remove from pan & set aside.
3. Place the saucepan back over low heat & melt the butter. Whisk in the flour & garlic. Continuously whisking, cook for 2 minutes.
4. Remove from heat. Whisk in the milk, nutmeg, salt & pepper. Return to heat & continue cooking until smooth.
5. Remove from heat. Stir in the egg yolks, swiss cheese & spinach mixture.
6. Whisk the egg whites & cream of tartar to firm peaks. Add a quarter of the egg whites to the yolk filling & stir to combine. Add the remaining egg whites & gently fold in, ensuring not to deflate the whites.
7. Evenly divide the mixture amongst the prepared ramekins. Place in the middle of the oven (removing the above racks) & turn heat down to 375(f) degrees.
8. Bake for 25 to 30 minutes, until puffed & golden. Do not peak until the 25 minute mark! Serve immediately.

Mushroom and Spinach Frittata

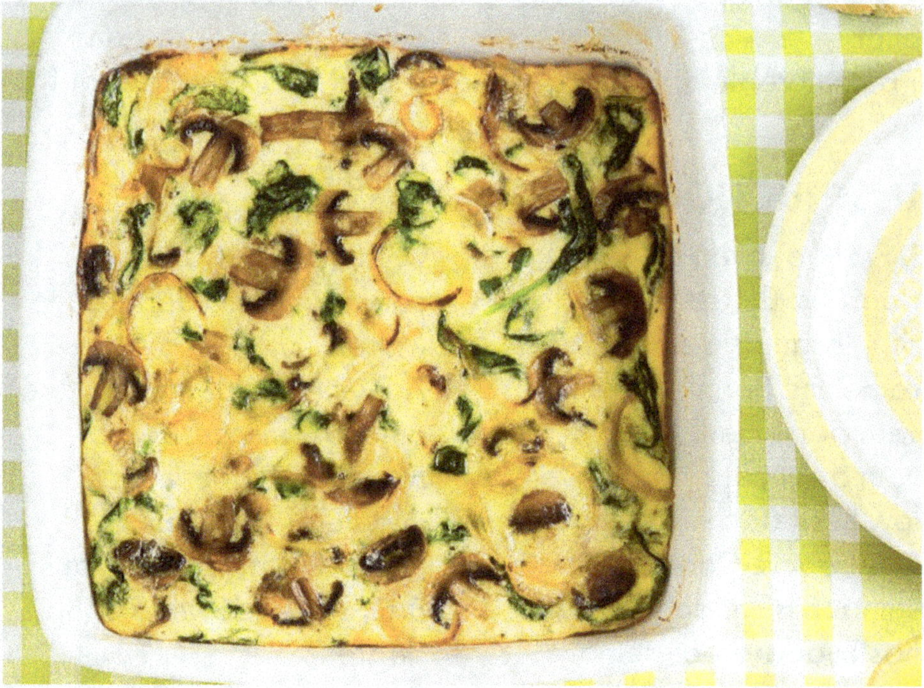

PREP
15 mins

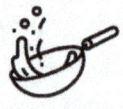
COOK
30 mins

SERVES
4

INGREDIENTS

6 eggs
1/4 cup (60 ml) milk
1 cup (250 ml) grated cheddar cheese
1 onion, thinly sliced
Salt and pepper
4 oz (115 g) white button mushrooms, sliced
3 tablespoons (45 ml) butter
2 cups (500 ml) baby spinach

INSTRUCTIONS

With the rack in the middle position, preheat the oven to 180 °C (350 °F). Butter a 20-cm (8-inch) square baking dish. Set aside.

In a large bowl, combine eggs and milk with a whisk. Add cheese. Season with salt and pepper. Place bowl aside.

In a large non-stick skillet, brown onion and mushrooms in butter over medium heat. Season with salt and pepper.

Add spinach and continue cooking for about 1 minute, stirring constantly.

Pour mushroom mixture into egg mixture. Stir well and pour into baking dish. Bake the frittata for about 25 minutes or until lightly browned and puffed. Cut frittata into four squares and remove from dish with a spatula. Place on a plate and voila, it is ready to serve warm or cold.

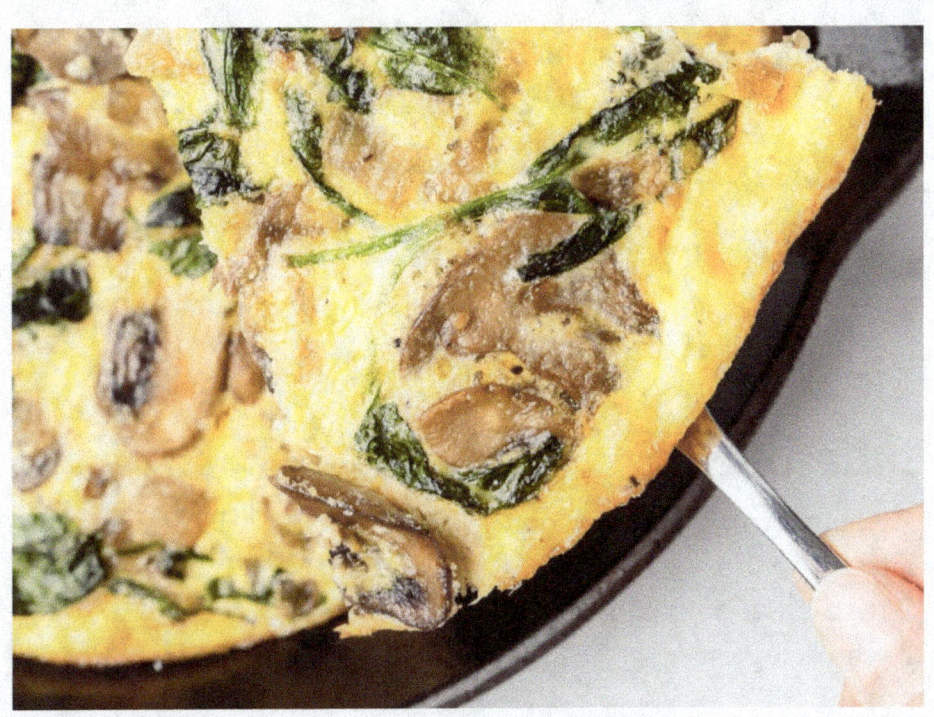

Baked Cod with Lemon and Capers

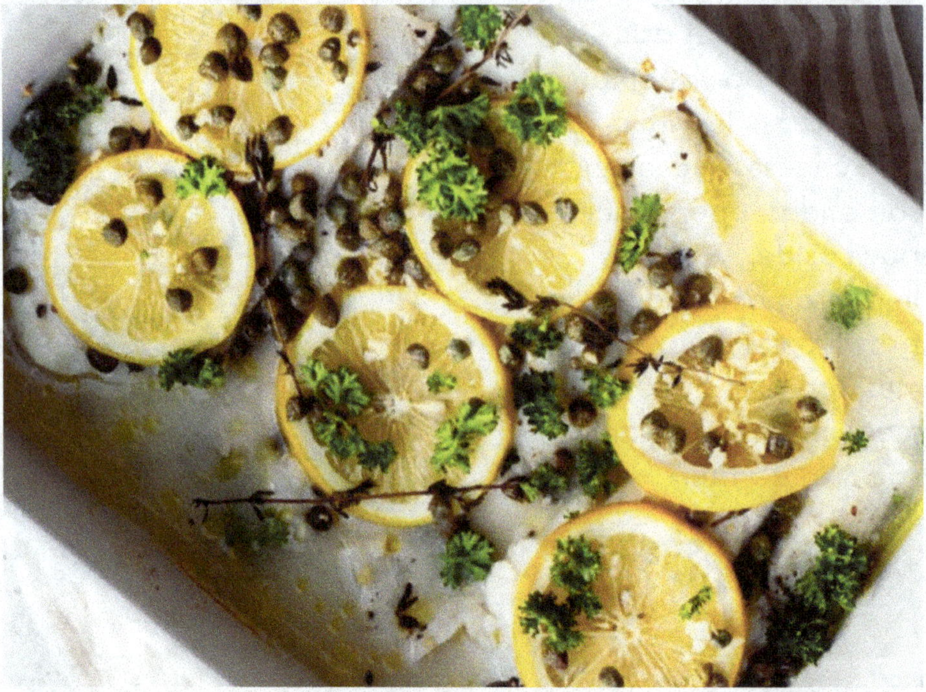

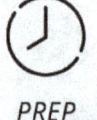
PREP
10 mins

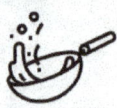
COOK
15 mins

SERVES
4

INGREDIENTS

2 pounds fresh cod fish, cut into 4 servings
2 tbsp olive oil, divided
2 whole lemons
Kosher salt
Pepper
2 tbsp capers drained from their liquid
2 tbsp fresh thyme leaves
2 cloves garlic, finely minced
Fresh parsley, for garnish

INSTRUCTIONS

Preheat the oven to 375 degrees F.

Arrange the cod fillets on a plate and drizzle with 1 tbsp olive oil, juice of 1 lemon, and a generous shake of salt and pepper. Let the cod marinate in this while the oven is heating up.

Transfer the cod to a 7.5" x 10.5" or 9" x 13" ceramic baking dish (it is fine if the pieces overlap a bit).

Top the cod with capers, fresh thyme, minced garlic, and remaining olive oil.

Slice the remaining lemon into rounds and arrange the slices on top of the cod. Add a few sprigs of fresh thyme if you have them.

Bake in the oven for 15-17 minutes, until fish is an internal temperature of 145 degrees F, and is opaque and flakes easily with a fork. Cook time will depend on the amount and thickness of fish.

Remove from oven and let sit for a minute or two before serving.

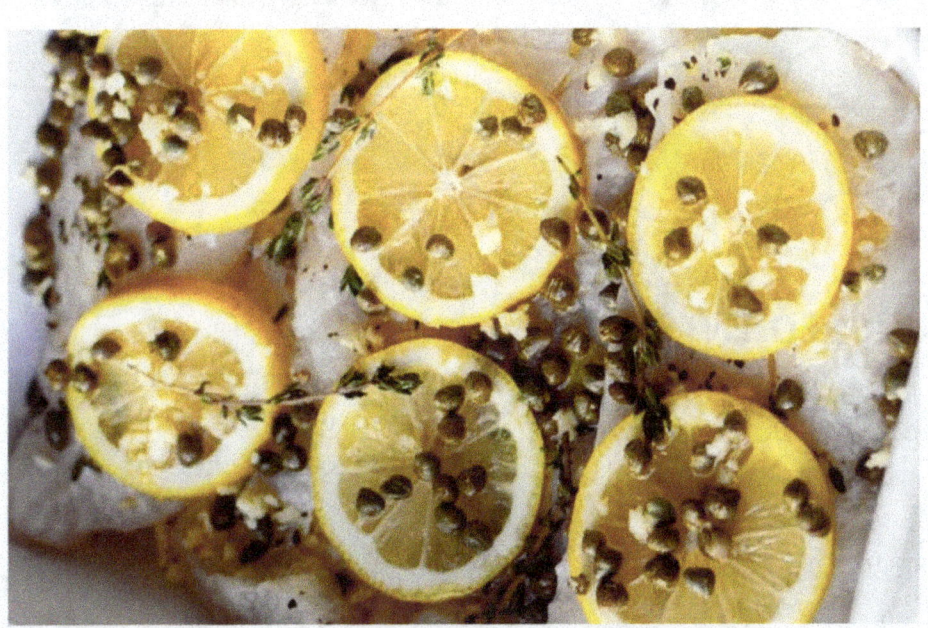

Veggie Pizza

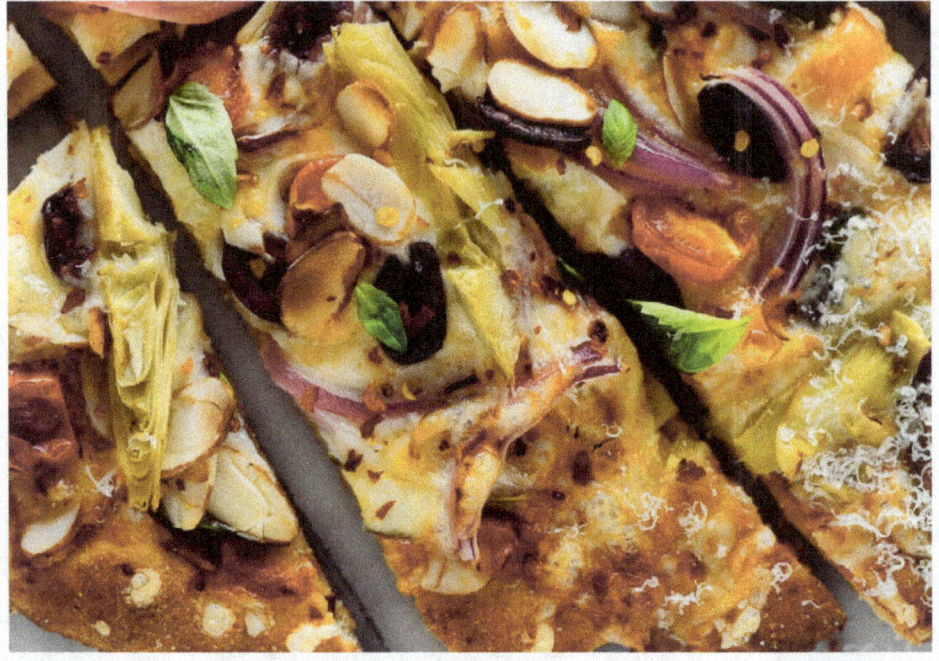

PREP
25 mins

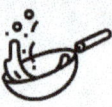
COOK
20 mins

SERVES
6

INGREDIENTS

1 batch easy whole wheat pizza dough or 1 pound store-bought pizza dough
1 cup pizza sauce or marinara
2 cups baby spinach

2 to 3 cups (8 to 12 ounces) shredded low-moisture part-skim mozzarella cheese
½ cup jarred or canned artichoke, cut into 1" pieces

½ cup fresh red or orange bell pepper, cut into narrow 2" strips
½ cup red onion, cut into thin wedges
½ cup halved cherry tomatoes
½ cup pitted Kalamata olives, halved lengthwise
½ cup sliced almonds (optional)
Optional garnishes: Fresh basil (small leaves or torn), red pepper flakes and/or finely grated Parmesan cheese

INSTRUCTIONS

Preheat the oven to 500 degrees Fahrenheit with a rack in the upper third of the oven. If you're using a baking stone or baking steel, place it on the upper rack. Prepare dough through step 5.

Spread pizza sauce evenly over the two pizzas, leaving about 1 inch bare around the edges.

Evenly distribute the spinach on top of the sauce, followed by the cheese

Top the pizzas with artichoke, bell pepper, red onion, tomatoes, olives and almonds (if using).

Bake pizzas individually on the top rack until the crust is golden and the cheese is golden and bubbly, about 10 to 12 minutes (or significantly less, if you're using a baking stone/steel—keep an eye on it).

Transfer pizzas to a cutting board and sprinkle with with fresh basil, red pepper flakes and Parmesan, if using. Slice and serve!

Leftover pizza keeps well in the refrigerator for 4 days, or for several months in the freezer.

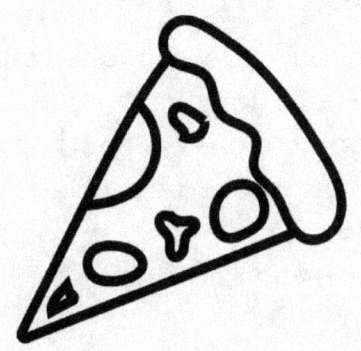

Grilled Shrimp Kabobs

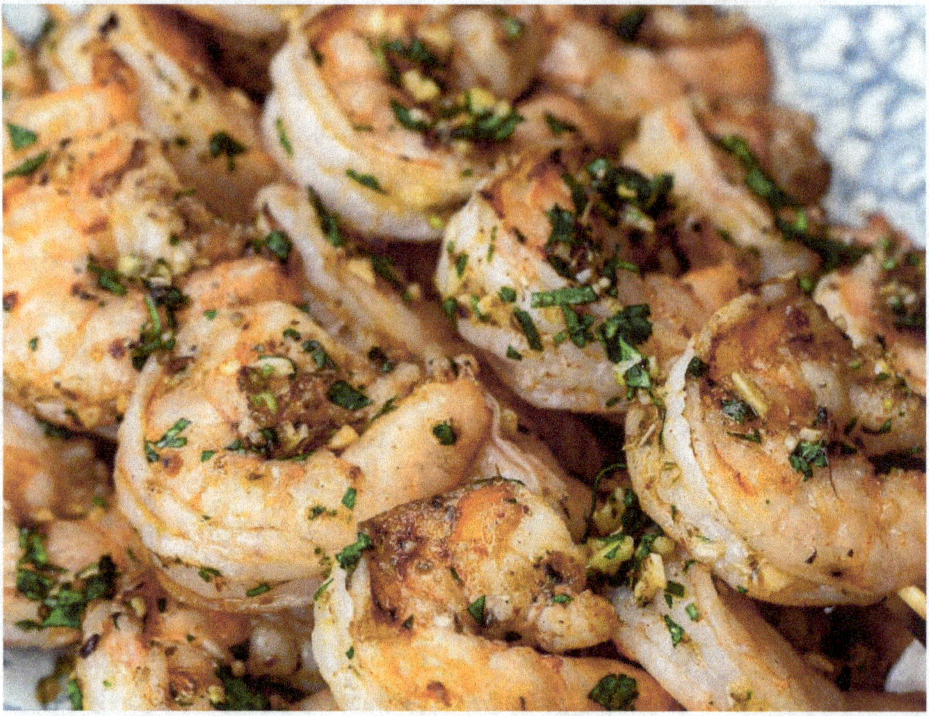

PREP
10 mins

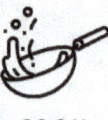

COOK
6 mins

SERVES
6

INGREDIENTS

⅓ cup Extra virgin olive oil
Zest of 2 lemons
4 garlic cloves minced
¼ cup packed chopped fresh parsley
1 teaspoon oregano
1 teaspoon paprika
½ teaspoon coriander
½ teaspoon red pepper flakes
2 lb large shrimp peeled and deveined
Kosher salt

INSTRUCTIONS

Combine the marinade ingredients in a small bowl. Reserve 2 tablespoon of the marinade in a separate bowl for later.

Pat the shrimp dry and season with kosher salt. Place the shrimp in a large bowl and pour the marinade all over. Toss to combine.

Cover and refrigerate for 20 to 30 minutes (do not go longer).

Thread the shrimp on skewers, about 4 large shrimp per skewer. (If using bamboo skewers they need to be soaked in water for at least 30 minutes first).

To grill on an outdoor gas grill. Preheat a gas grill to high. Then, reduce heat to low (temperature should be somewhere between 275 to 325°F). Carefully grease the cooking grates. Once the grill reaches the recommended temperature, add the shrimp skewers and close the lid.

Cook shrimp for 2 to 3 minutes on each side or until no longer translucent.

To grill on an indoor griddle or cast iron grill. Heat a dry griddle over medium-high heat until hot but not smoking. Add the shrimp skewers and cook on one side about 3 or 4 minutes. Turn shrimp over and cook another 2 to 3 minutes.

Transfer the grilled shrimp skewers to platter and spoon the remaining marinade your reserved earlier over the grilled shrimp skewers. Add a splash of lemon juice. Serve immediately.

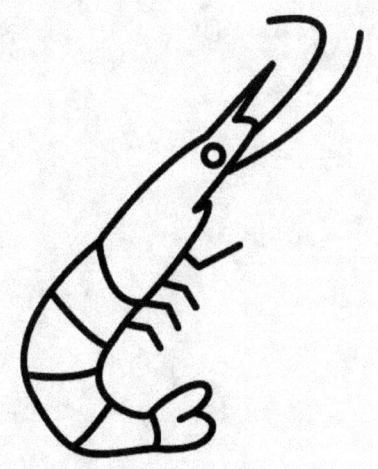

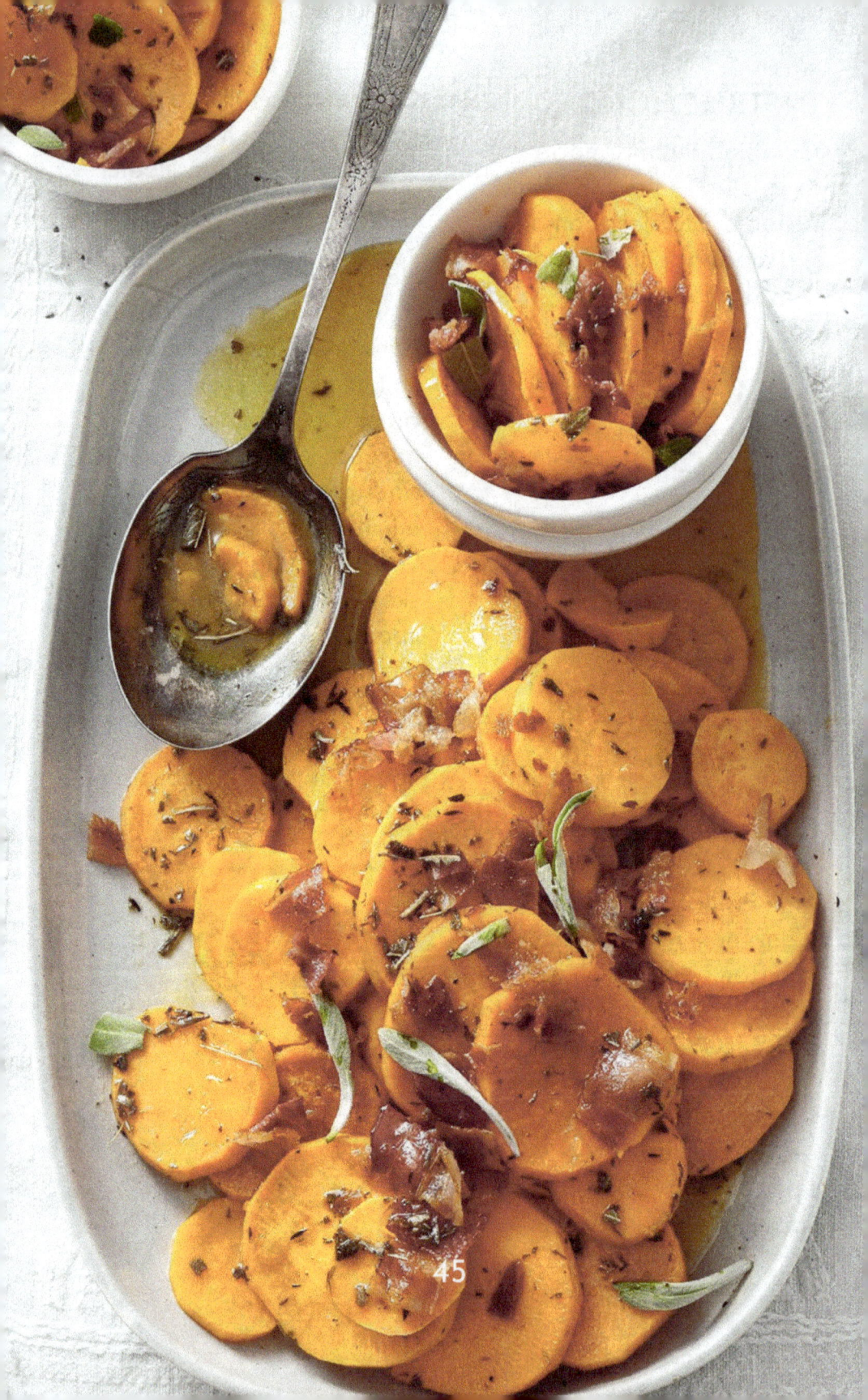

SIDE DISH

Green Bean Casserole

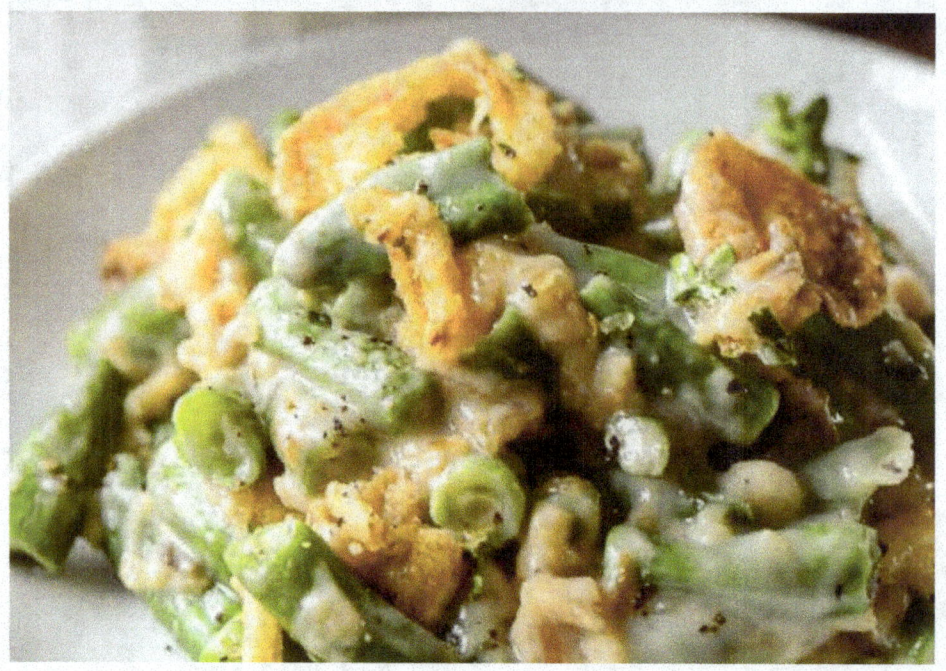

PREP
10 mins

COOK
40 mins

SERVES
8

INGREDIENTS

4 cups frozen cut green bean defrosted (see notes for canned or fresh beans)

10 ½ ounces cream of mushroom soup

½ cup milk

1 teaspoon soy sauce

¼ teaspoon seasoning salt or to taste

1 ½ cups crispy fried onions divided

½ teaspoon black pepper

INSTRUCTIONS

Preheat oven to 350°F. If using fresh or frozen green beans, boil just until tender crisp. (see note) Combine green beans with soup, milk, soy sauce, pepper, salt, 1 cup of crispy onions, and cheese (if using, see note) in a casserole dish.

Bake uncovered for 30-35 minutes or bubbly. Remove from oven and stir. Top with remaining onions and return to oven for an additional 10 minutes or until golden.

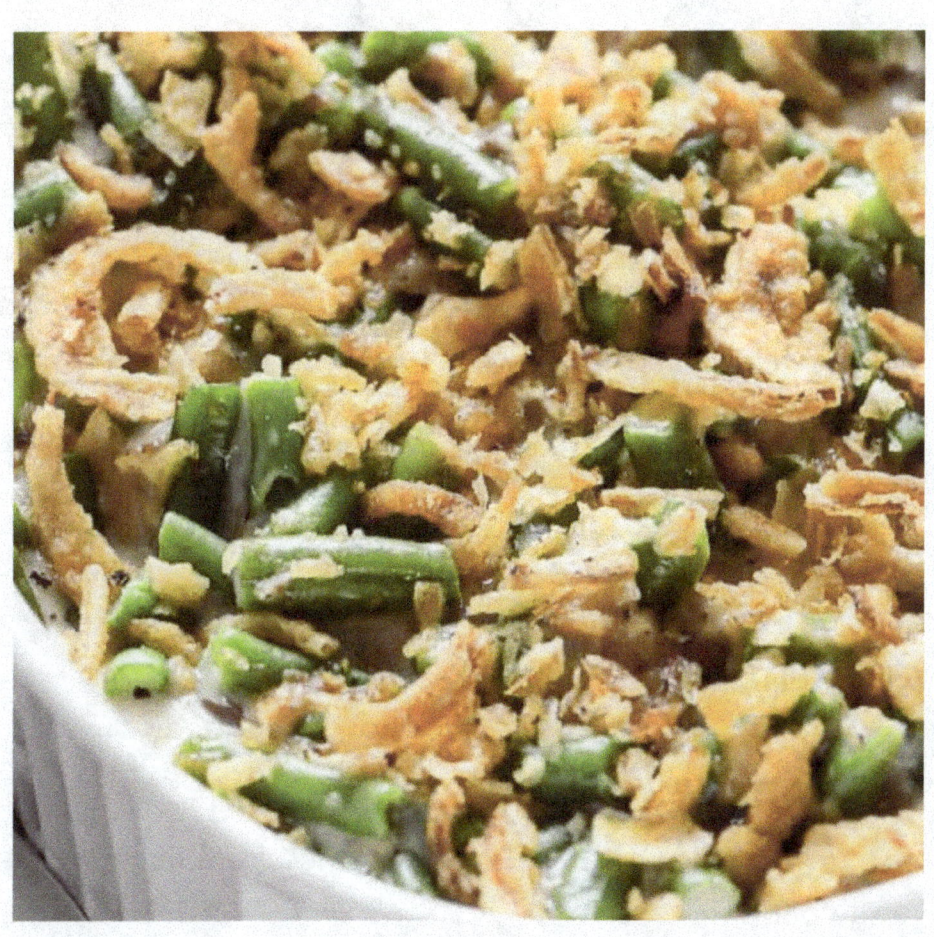

Honey Roasted Carrots with Sage

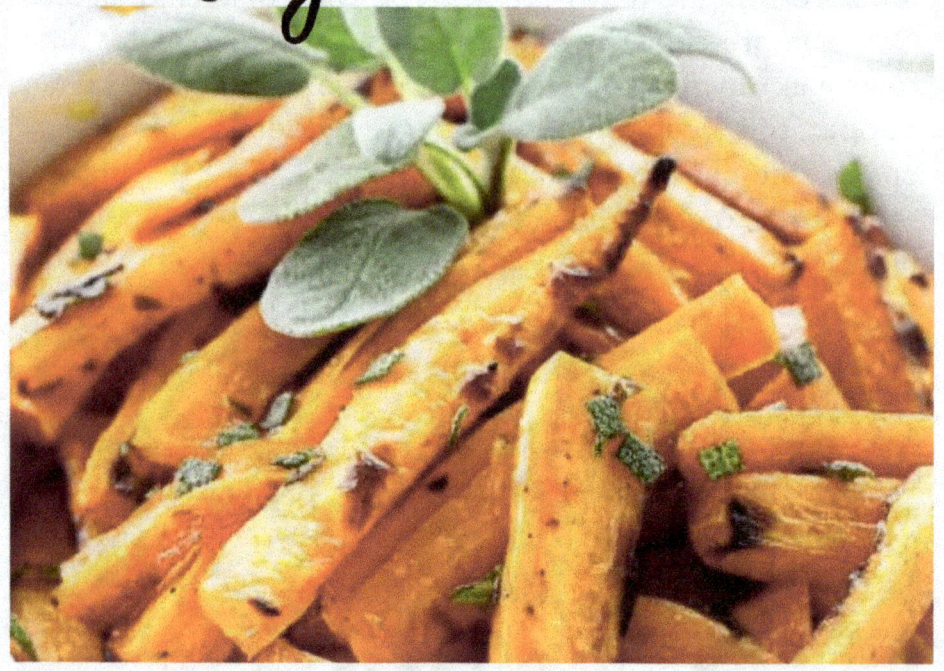

PREP
10 mins

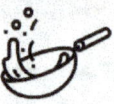
COOK
15 mins

SERVES
8

INGREDIENTS

3 pounds carrots
2 tablespoons extra virgin olive oil
½ teaspoon freshly ground white pepper
1 teaspoon fresh sage leaves chopped
Fresh sage sprigs for garnish
3 tablespoons honey
1 teaspoon sea salt

INSTRUCTIONS

Preheat the oven to 450°F. Line a sheet pan with parchment paper and set aside.

Wash the carrots under cold water then peel them and cut lengthwise into quarters, then in 3-inch sections. Place the carrots in a large bowl, and toss with the olive oil, honey, salt, pepper, and chopped sage.

Spread the carrots in a single layer onto the prepared sheet pan. Transfer to the oven and roast for 15 minutes until the carrots are tender and begin to caramelize. Remove the pan from the oven and transfer the carrots to a serving dish. Garnish with chopped fresh sage and sage sprigs. Serve hot.

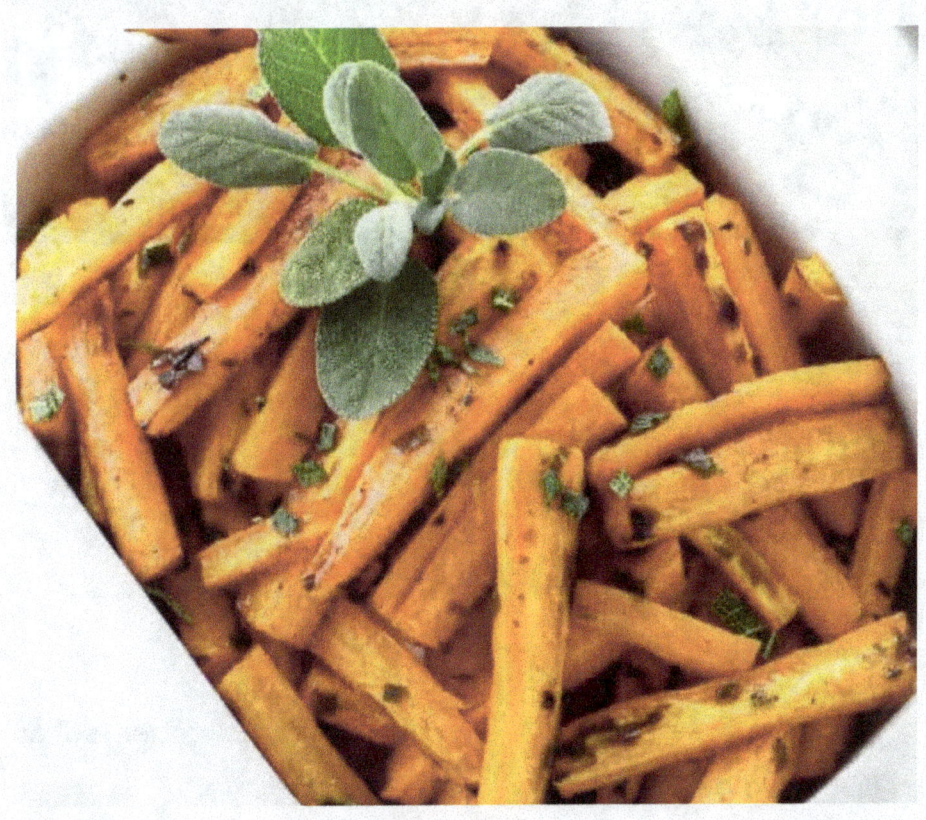

Lemony Fava Beans with Garlic and Cilantro

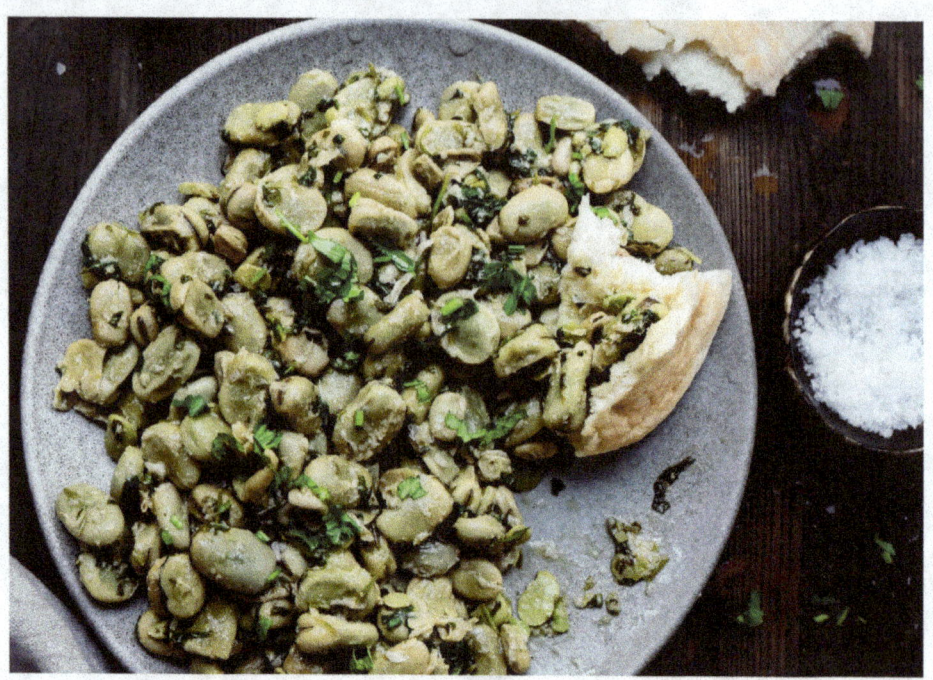

PREP
10 mins

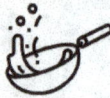
COOK
10 mins

SERVES
4

INGREDIENTS

1 kg/2 lbs shelled fava beans, fresh or frozen (about 2.6 kg/5 lb fresh with pods)
1/2 c olive oil
1 head garlic
1 tsp salt, plus more to taste
2 c chopped cilantro/coriander leaves
1-2 lemons

INSTRUCTIONS

Boil the fava beans until the skin easily pierces with your fingernail. This will vary depending on the beans, 1-15 minutes, fresh tends to need longer. Transfer to an ice bath or a medium-sized bowl.

In a large skillet set over medium-low heat, add olive oil, garlic, salt and fava beans. Cook, stirring frequently, until fully cooked through and flavorful, about 10-15 minutes. If at any point the garlic or fava beans are sticking to the pan, add 1/4 c of water to deglaze.

Remove from the heat and stir in the cilantro/coriander leaves. Squeeze lemon over the top, combine, and adjust seasoning.

Transfer to a serving platter to marinade the flavors and cool completely. You can also reserve in an airtight container and serve the next day. Take it out of the fridge 30-60 minutes ahead of time to allow to come to room temperature. Serve with pita bread.

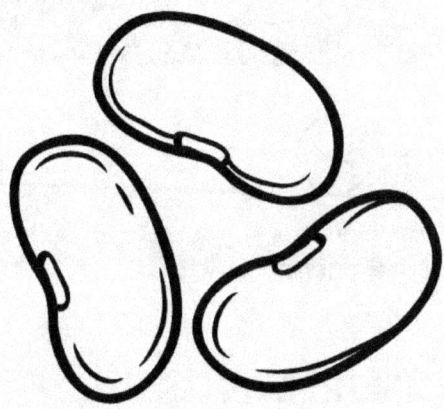

Spicy Snow Peas

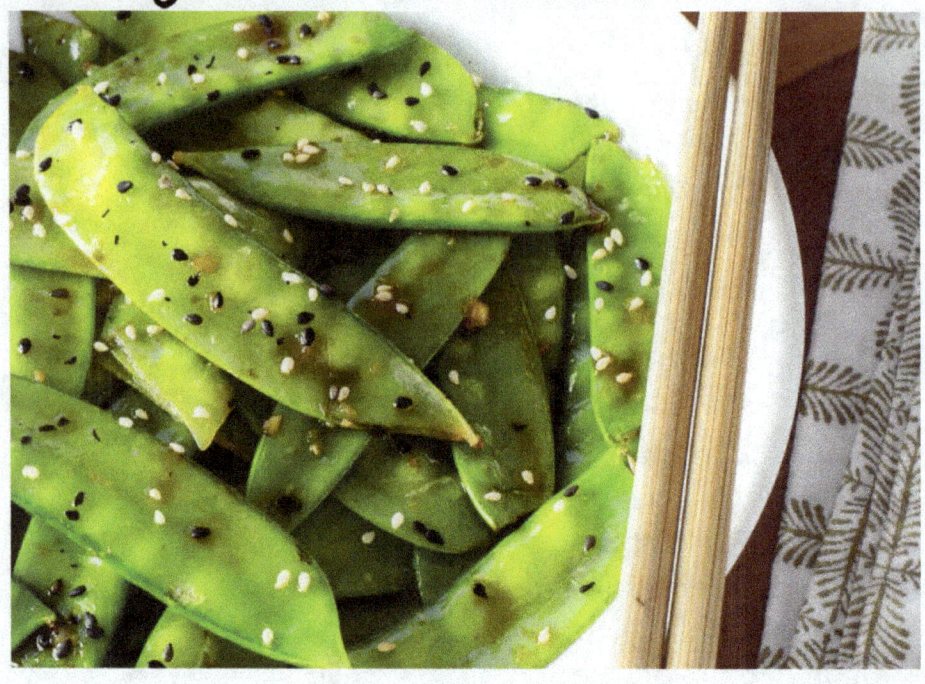

PREP
5 mins

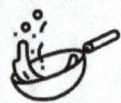
COOK
5 mins

SERVES
4

INGREDIENTS

1½ tsp sesame oil
1 tsp chili oil *Click the link up above for the recipe
8 oz snow peas
½ tsp fresh ginger, grated
1 clove of garlic, minced

Sea salt and freshly cracked pepper, to taste
Toasted sesame seeds or black sesame seeds, optional

INSTRUCTIONS

Heat the sesame oil and the chili oil together in a large saute pan.

Add the snow peas and toss to coat evenly. Cook, stirring often, for 3 minutes.

Add the minced ginger and garlic and cook, stirring constantly, for 1 minute.

Season the sesame snow peas with sea salt and freshly cracked pepper, to taste.

Pour into a serving bowl and sprinkle with toasted sesame seeds, black sesame seeds, or both, to taste.

Serve immediately with additional chili oil and some soy sauce on the side, if desired. Enjoy.

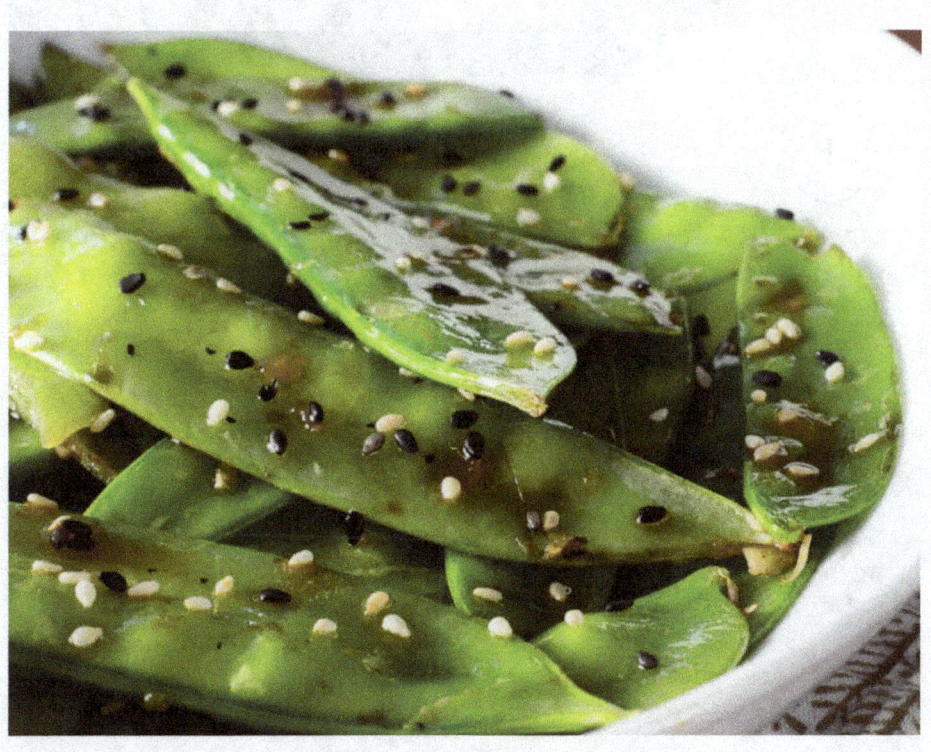

Oven Roasted Beets

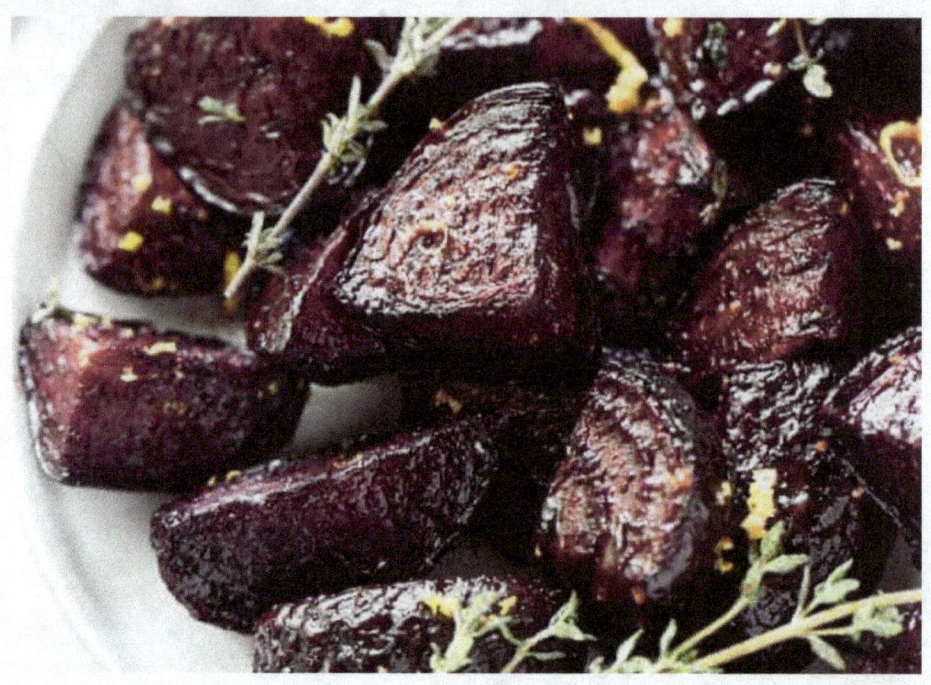

PREP
15 mins

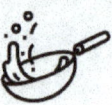
COOK
40 mins

SERVES
4

INGREDIENTS

3 large beets, (can also use 4 medium beets or 5 small beets)
1 tablespoon extra virgin olive oil

1 teaspoon kosher salt
1/2 teaspoon freshly ground black pepper
1 teaspoon orange zest
1 teaspoon fresh thyme leaves, minced

Lemony Seared Endives

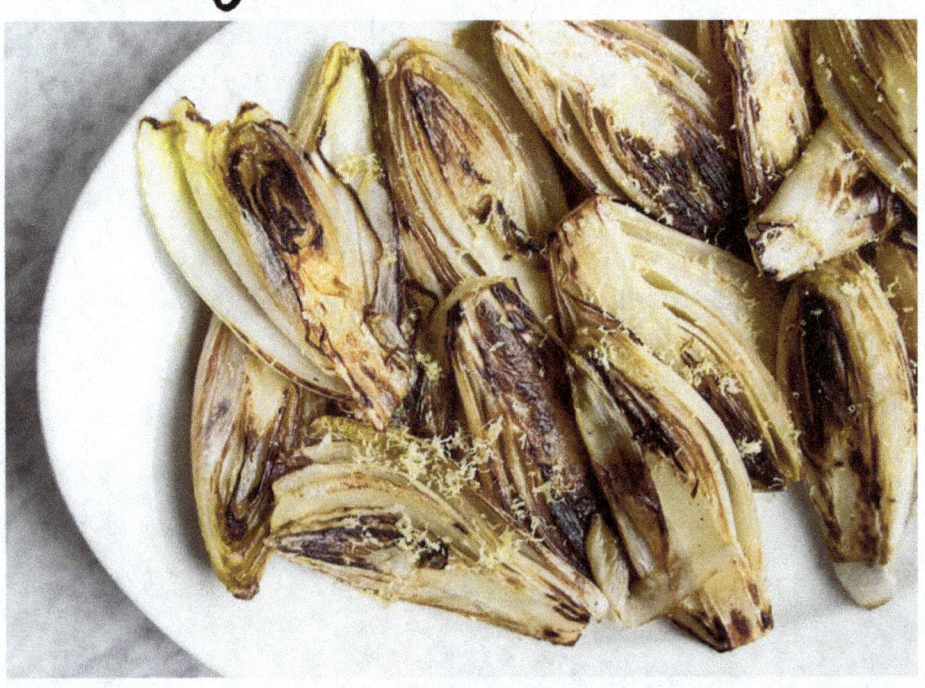

PREP
20 mins

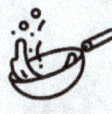
COOK
10 mins

SERVES
8

INGREDIENTS

4 ½ tablespoons extra-virgin olive oil (plus more for drizzling)
8 Belgian endives (large halved lengthwise)
Kosher salt

1 tablespoon lemon zest (plus fresh lemon juice finely grated)
Flaky sea salt (for sprinkling)

INSTRUCTIONS

In a large skillet, heat 1 1/2 tablespoons of the olive oil until shimmering. Add one-third of the halved endives; season with kosher salt. Cook over moderately high heat, turning once, until browned and starting to soften, about 3 minutes; transfer to a platter.

Repeat in 2 more batches with the remaining olive oil and endives. Top with the lemon zest and juice, drizzle with more olive oil and sprinkle with sea salt. Serve immediately.

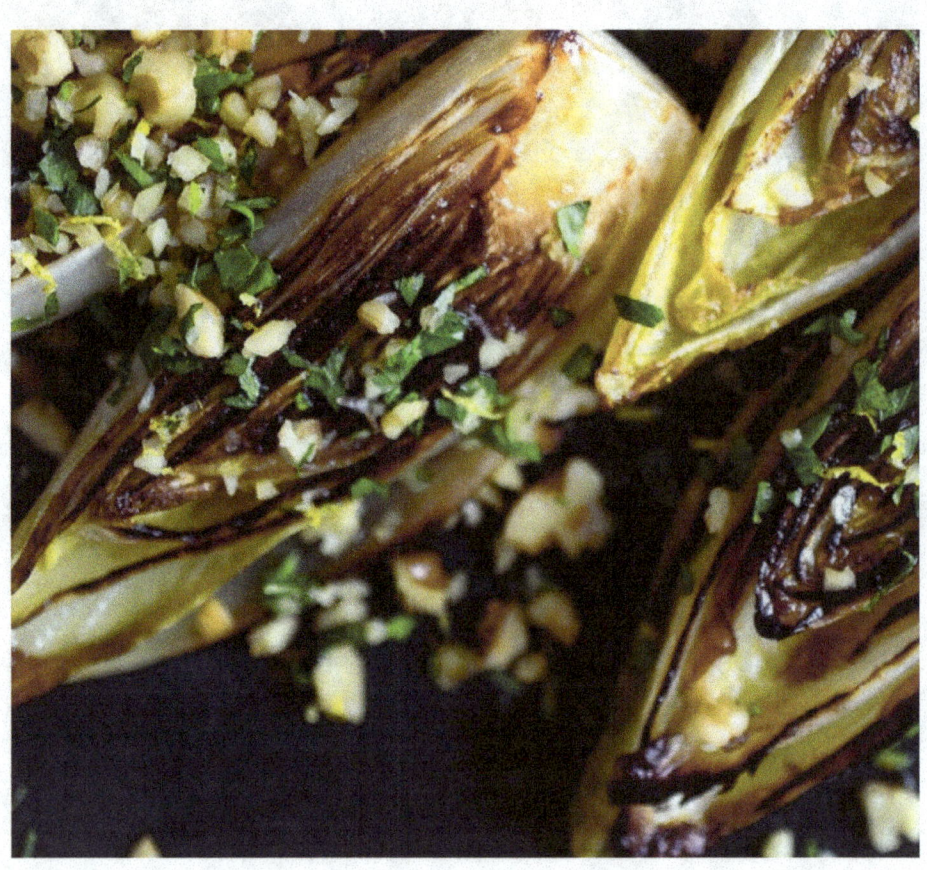

Braised Kale And Tomatoes

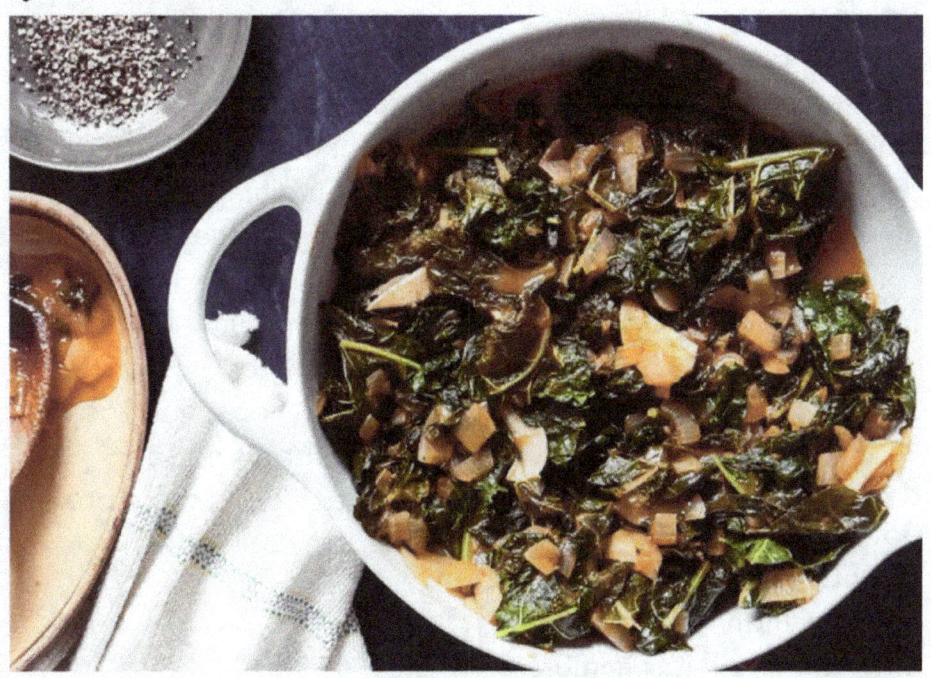

PREP
20 mins

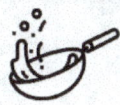
COOK
40 mins

SERVES
8-10

INGREDIENTS

¼cup extra-virgin olive oil
2 Spanish onions, peeled and diced
8 cloves garlic, peeled and thinly sliced
¼cup tomato paste
1 teaspoon hot smoked paprika (pimentón)
Kosher salt and freshly ground black pepper, to taste

3 cups turkey or chicken stock, ideally homemade or low-sodium
1 tablespoon red wine vinegar, plus more to taste
4 (¾-pound) bunches washed kale (any kind), thick stems discarded or cut into thin strips, leaves cut into thick strips (about 16 packed cups total)

INSTRUCTIONS

Place a large, heavy-bottomed, high-sided pot or Dutch oven over medium-high heat and add olive oil. When it shimmers, add onions and garlic and cook until they soften and begin to turn translucent, about 5 to 7 minutes. Add tomato paste and smoked paprika, reduce heat to medium, and cook, stirring frequently, until the paste begins to caramelize, about 5 to 7 minutes. Season with salt and pepper, then add stock and vinegar, and allow to come to a boil.
Add half the kale, cover, and cook for a minute or two, until it wilts. Repeat with remaining kale. Stir to incorporate the onion mixture into the soft kale and simmer until tender, 20 to 30 minutes, partly covered. Season to taste with salt and pepper, drizzle with a little more vinegar, and serve.

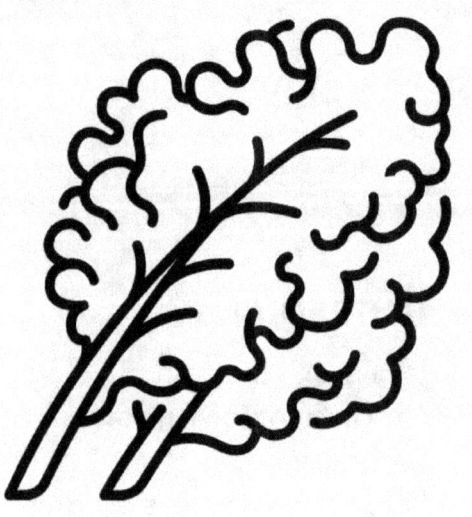

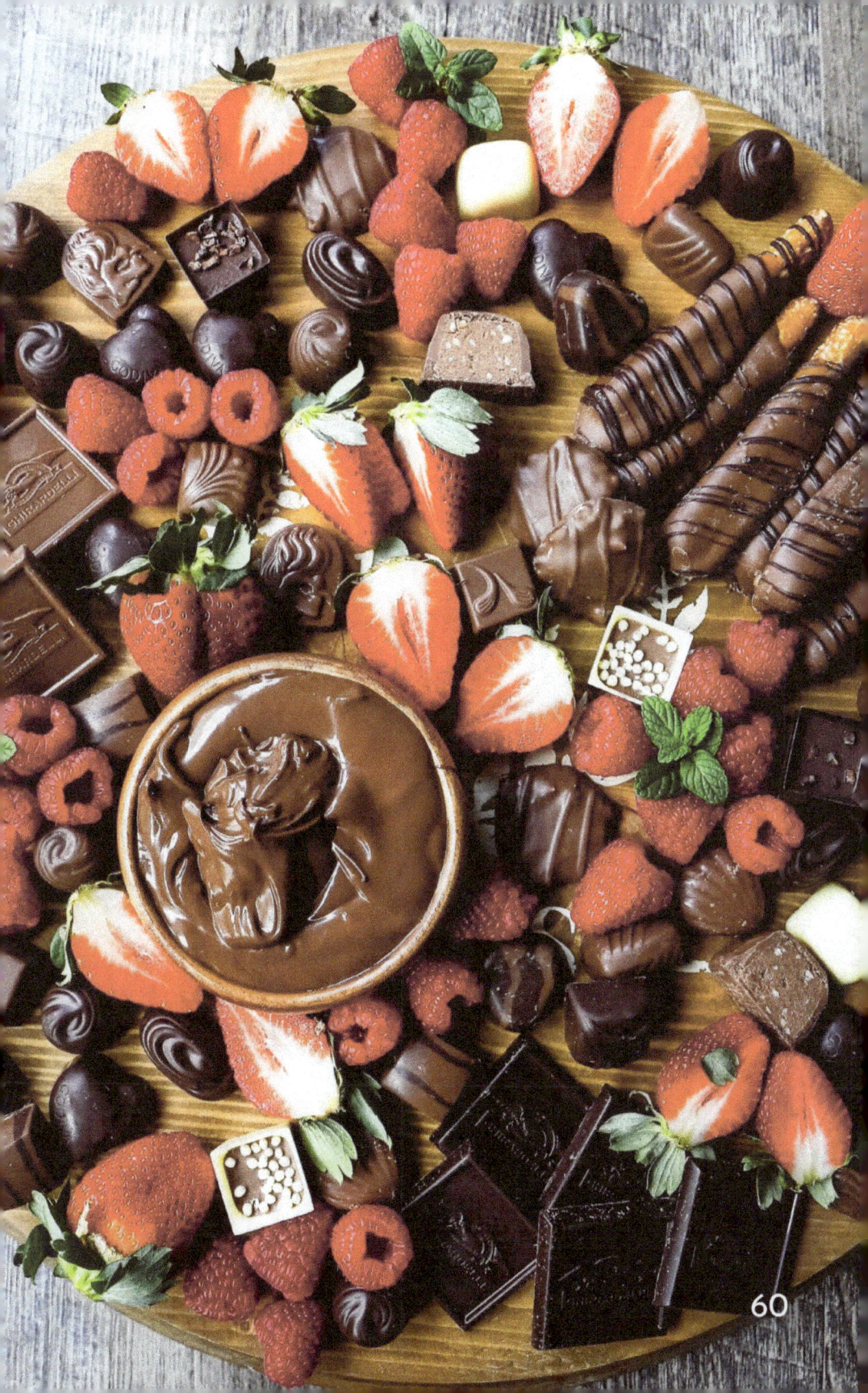

DESSERT

Moist Chocolate Cake

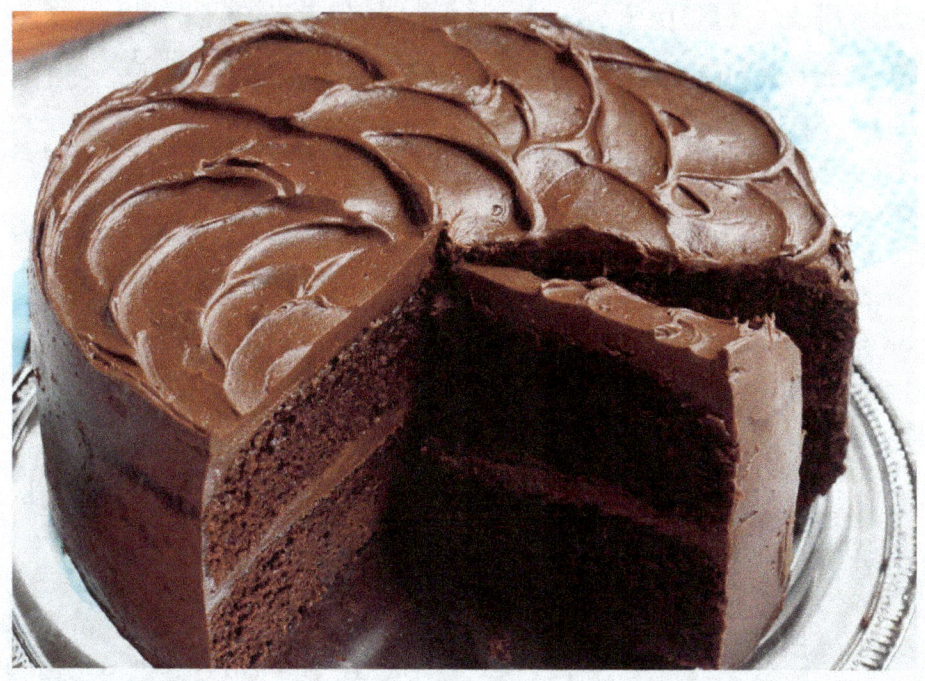

PREP
15 mins

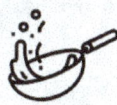
COOK
35 mins

SERVES
10

INGREDIENTS

1 ¾ cup 250g all-purpose flour
⅔ cup 56g cocoa powder (I prefer this one)
1 teaspoon baking powder
1 teaspoon baking soda
1 cup 200g granulated sugar
2 large eggs
½ cup 110g packed light brown sugar
¾ teaspoon salt
½ cup 120ml vegetable oil (I prefer sunflower oil)
¾ cup 180ml sour cream
1 teaspoon 5ml pure vanilla extract
1 cup 240ml hot coffee

INSTRUCTIONS

Preheat oven to 350°F. Lightly grease and flour two 8-inch round cake pans and line the base with rounds of parchment paper.

Sift flour, cocoa, baking powder and baking soda into a large bowl. Add both sugars and salt and whisk to blend well, pressing out any lumps of brown sugar. Combine eggs, oil, sour cream and vanilla in a medium bowl and whisk to blend well. Pour into the bowl with the dry ingredients and mix with an electric hand mixer on medium-low until blended. It will be thick and somewhat dry. Add the hot coffee gradually in two stages to minimize clumps forming and beat until evenly combined and the batter smooth.

Divide batter evenly between the prepared pans and bake for 30-33 minutes until cakes spring back when pressed gently and a skewer inserted into the center comes out clean. Transfer pans to a wire rack and let cool for 15 minutes before inverting onto the rack to cool completely.

Assemble the cake. Once cakes are cooled, place one cake layer on a serving plate. Use an offset spatula to spread about ¾ cup of frosting over the top, spreading it out to the edges. Place the other cake layer on top so it aligns with the sides of the bottom layer. Cover the entire cake with frosting and use the offset spatula to even out the sides and make swooshes and swirls on the top layer. Enjoy!

Rhubarb Pecan Muffins

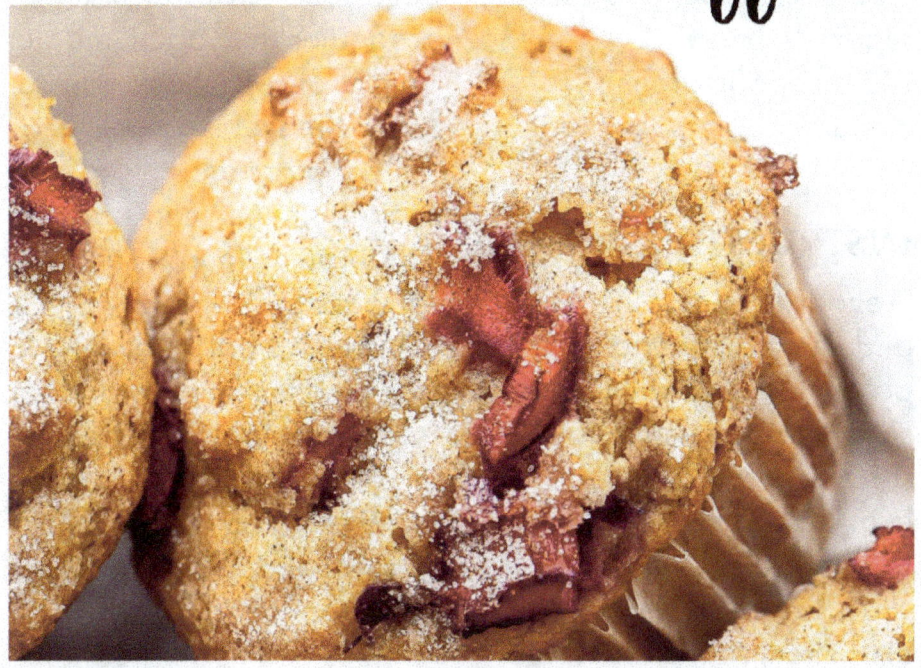

PREP
15 mins

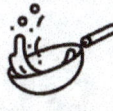
COOK
17 mins

SERVES
12-14

INGREDIENTS

2 cups white whole wheat flour
1 1/2 teaspoons ground cinnamon
1 teaspoon baking powder
1/2 teaspoon baking soda
1/2 teaspoon kosher salt
1/3 cup toasted pecans, chopped
1 1/2 cups diced rhubarb
1 cup plain non fat Greek yogurt
1/2 cup maple syrup
1/4 cup avocado oil or melted coconut oil
2 eggs
1 1/2 teaspoons vanilla extract

2 tablespoons granulated sugar
1/2 teaspoon ground cinnamon

INSTRUCTIONS

Preheat oven to 400° F. and line a muffin pan with parchment paper liners or spray the pan with cooking spray.

In a large bowl whisk together the flour, baking soda, baking powder, cinnamon, salt, pecans, and rhubarb

In a second bowl whisk together the yogurt, maple syrup, oil, eggs, and vanilla. Pour the wet ingredients into the dry and fold together until incorporated and you no longer see streaks of flour.

Divide the batter evenly into the muffin cups and top with some of the cinnamon sugar. Bake for 15-18 minutes or until golden brown and a toothpick inserted in the center comes out clean. Cool the muffins on a wire rack.

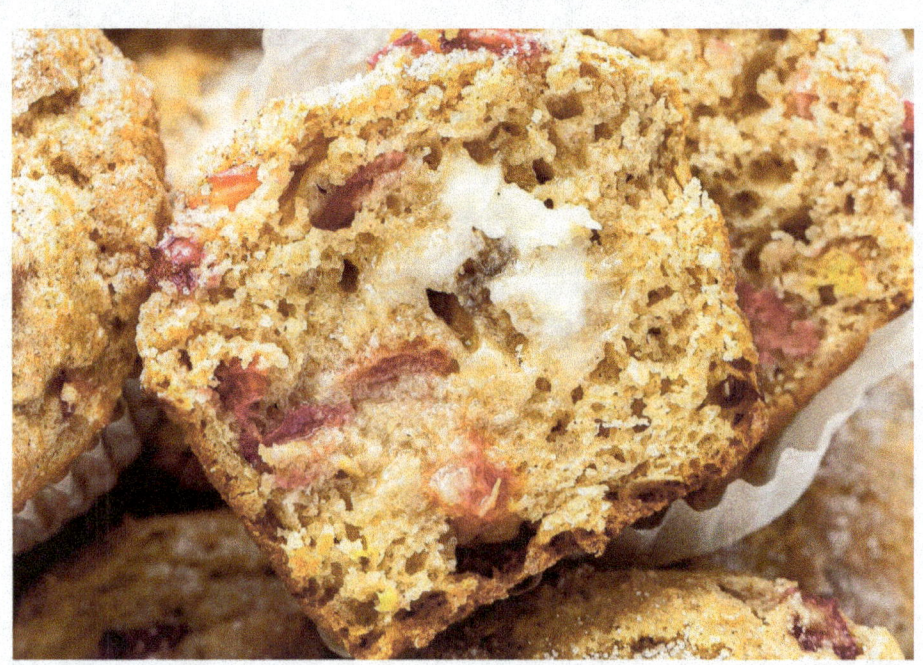

Lemon Cheesecake

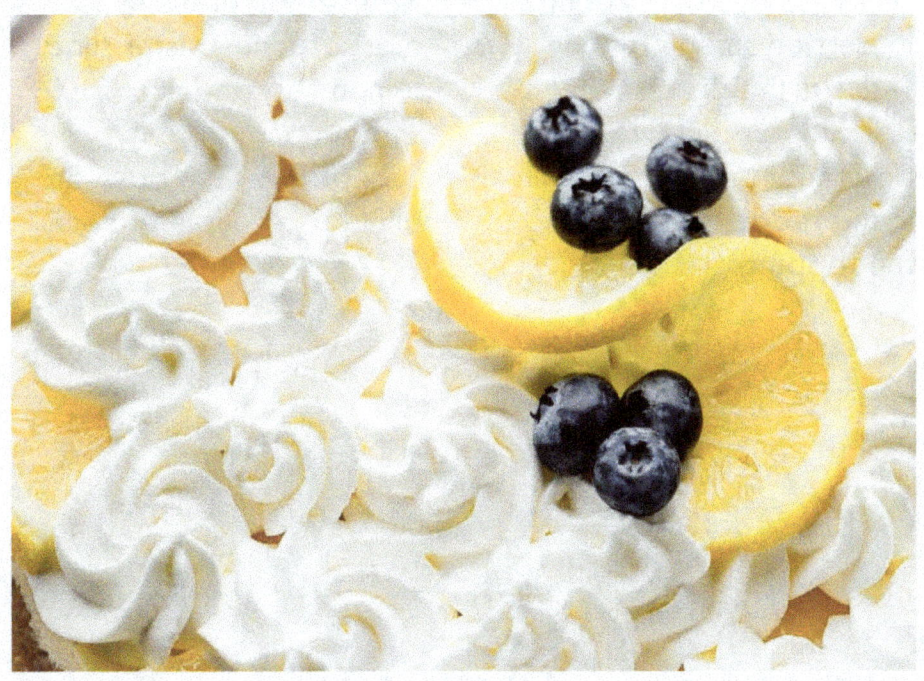

PREP
1 hour

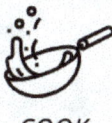

COOK
1 hour

SERVES
16

INGREDIENTS

110g digestive biscuits
50g butter
25g light brown soft sugar
350g mascarpone
75g caster sugar
1 lemon, zested
2-3 lemons, juiced (about 90ml)

INSTRUCTIONS

Crush the digestive biscuits in a food bag with a rolling pin or in the food processor. Melt the butter in a saucepan, take off heat and stir in the brown sugar and biscuit crumbs.

Line the base of a 20cm loose bottomed cake tin with baking parchment. Press the biscuit into the bottom of the tin and chill in the fridge while making the topping.

Beat together the mascarpone, caster sugar, lemon zest and juice, until smooth and creamy. Spread over the base and chill for a couple of hours.

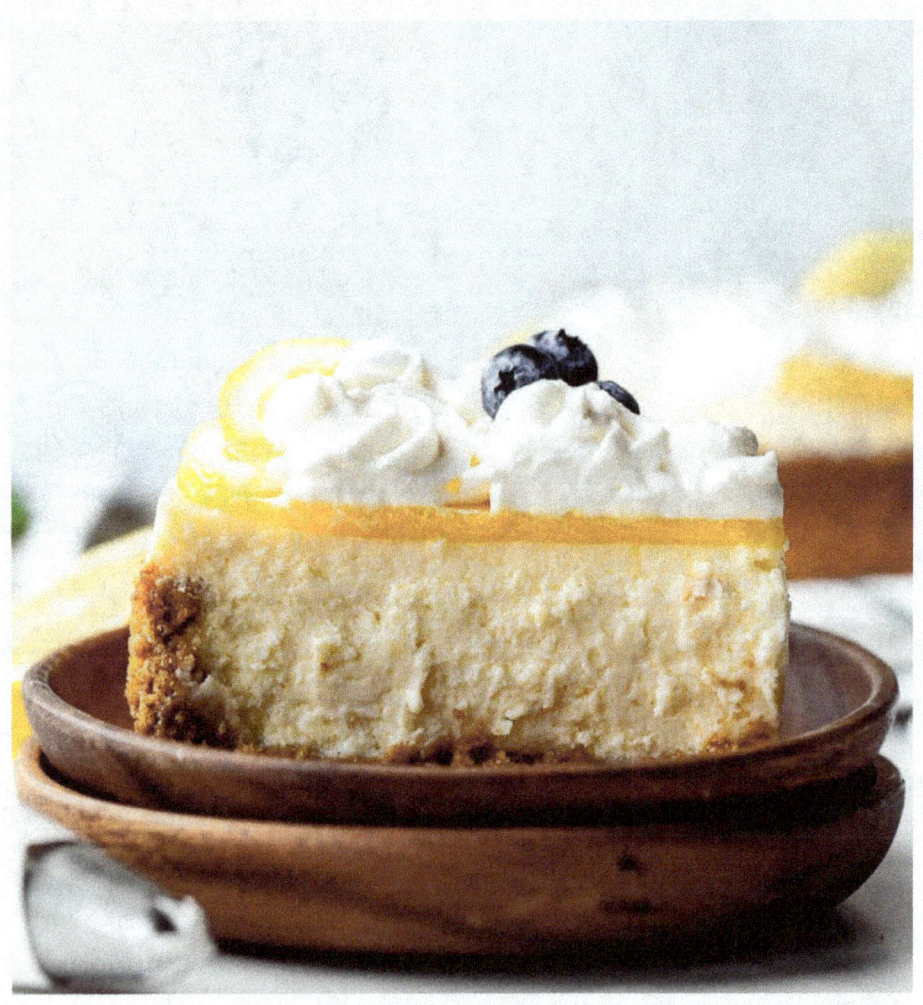

Fruit and Nut Bars

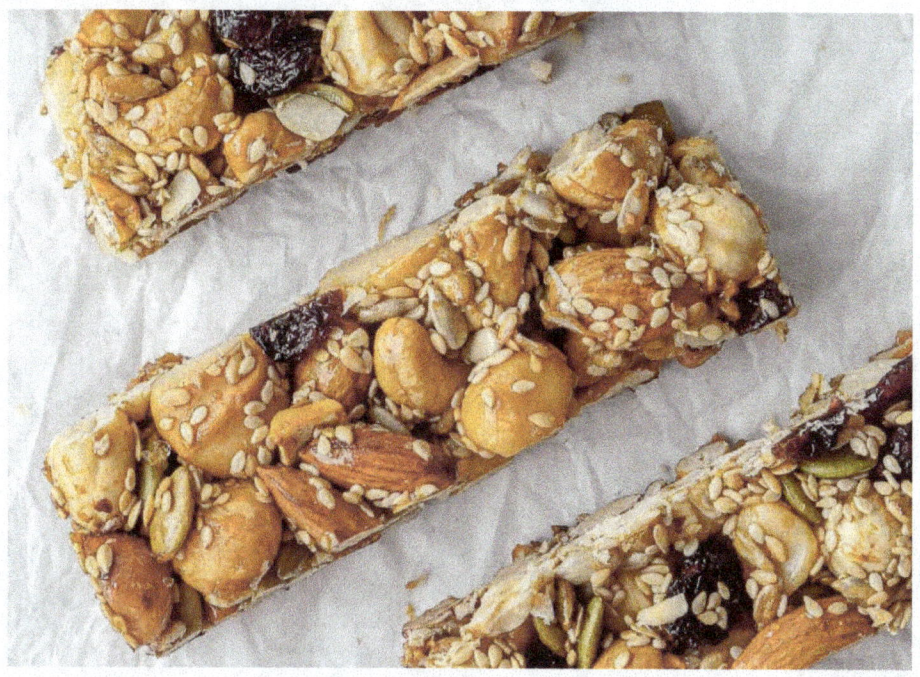

PREP
5 mins

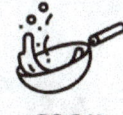
COOK
40 mins

SERVES
12 bars

INGREDIENTS

1 cup whole nuts, you can use cashews, walnuts, pecans, almonds, macadamia nuts.
1 cup chopped nuts, you can use cashews, walnuts, pecans, almonds, macadamia nuts.
½ cup dried cranberries
¼ cup sunflower seeds
¼ cup pumpkin seeds
¼ cup sesame seeds
1 Tbsp flaxseeds
½ tsp salt
½ cup honey
2 tsp vanilla extract

INSTRUCTIONS

Preheat oven to 350 degrees F. Spray with cooking spray and line an 8" square baking pan with parchment paper.

Place all the ingredients into a large bowl and mix them thoroughly.

Transfer the mixture to the baking pan. With the help of the spatula flatten the nuts down in one layer by firmly pressing on them.

Bake anywhere from 30-40 minutes until the nuts start to brown a little. They will have a nice deep golden-brown color.

Cool the bars in the pan completely. For about 2-3 hrs. Transfer to a cutting board and cut into 12 bars. Wrap each bar individually in parchment paper. Store in the refrigerator for 1 week or freeze for longer storage.

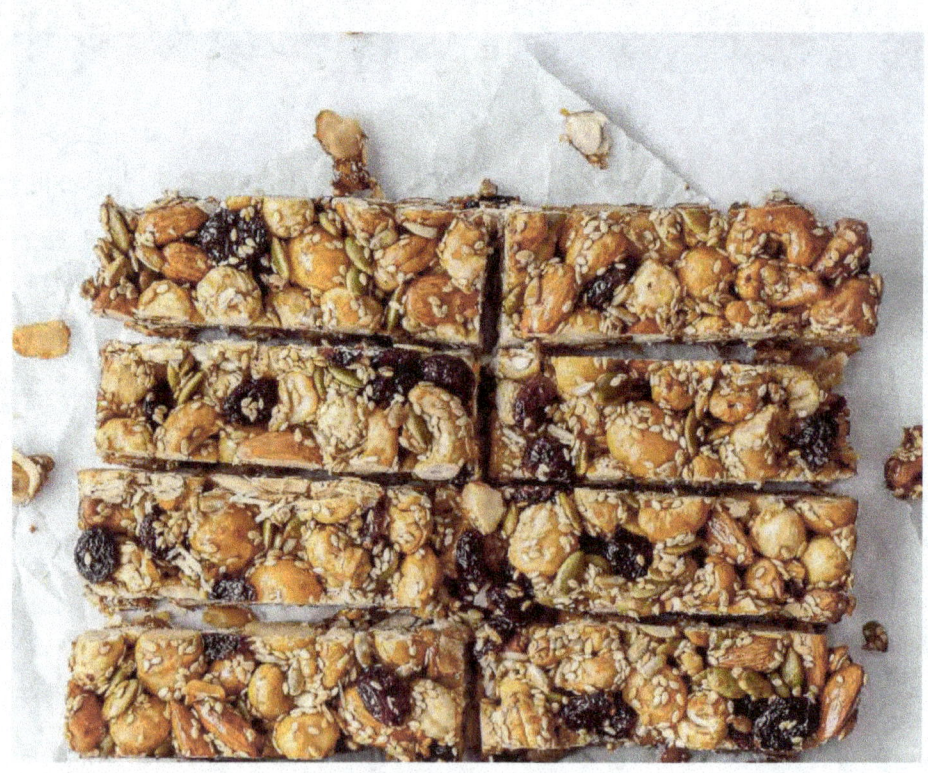

Easy Red, White, and Blue Parfaits

PREP
10 mins

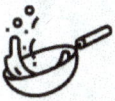
COOK
5 mins

SERVES
6

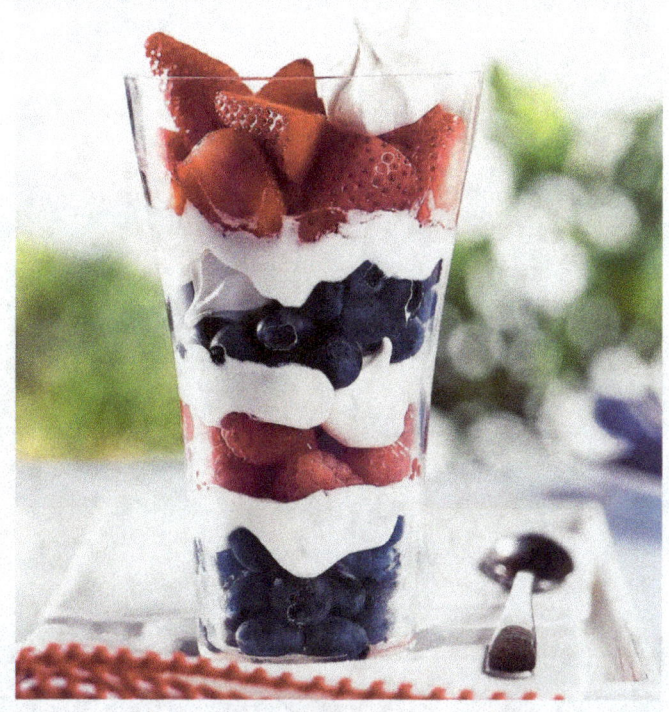

INGREDIENTS

¼ teaspoon almond extract or 1/2 teaspoon vanilla

½ 8 ounce container frozen light whipped dessert topping, thawed

3 cup fresh raspberries and/or cut-up fresh strawberries

3 cup fresh blueberries

1 8 ounce carton vanilla low-fat yogurt

INSTRUCTIONS

In a large bowl, stir together yogurt and almond extract or vanilla. Fold in whipped topping.

To serve, in six 12-ounce glasses or dessert dishes, alternate layers of the berries with layers of the yogurt mixture. Makes 6 servings.

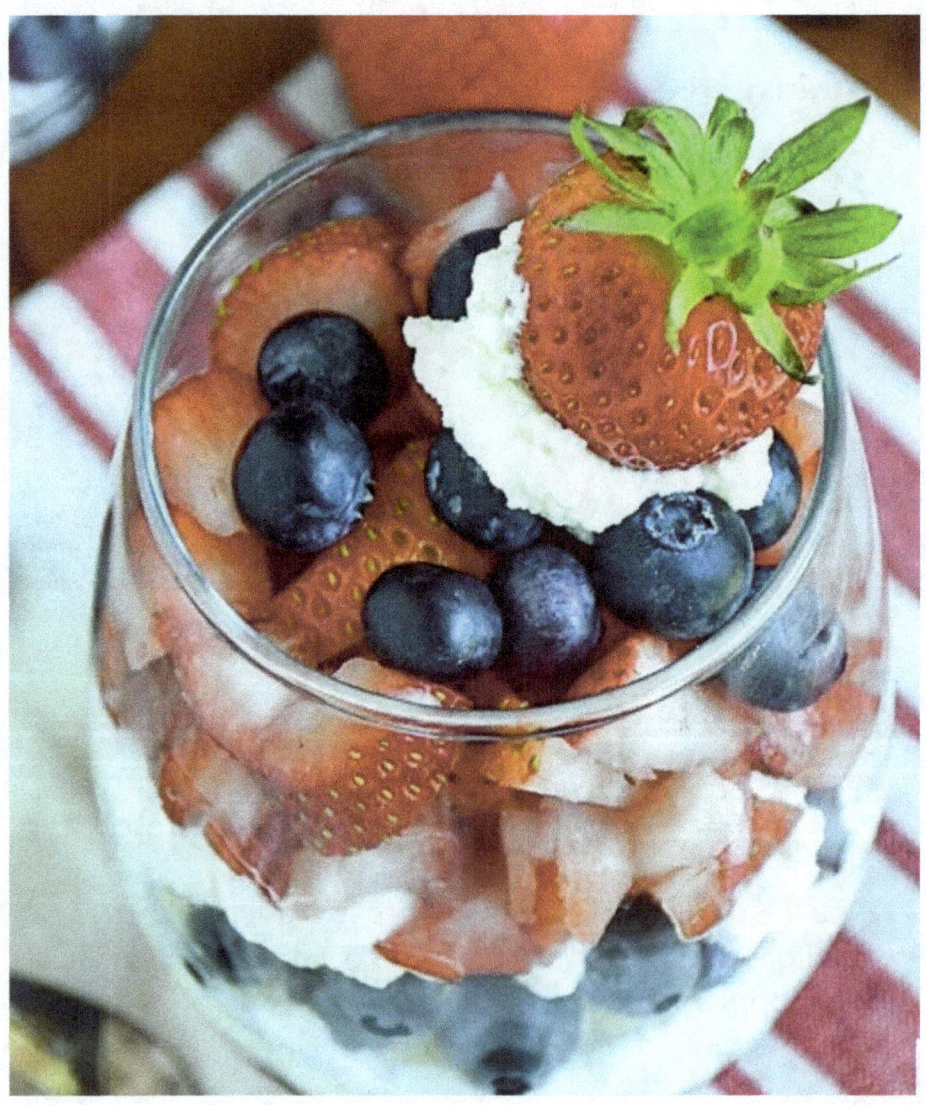

Rice Pudding with Honey Soaked Fruit

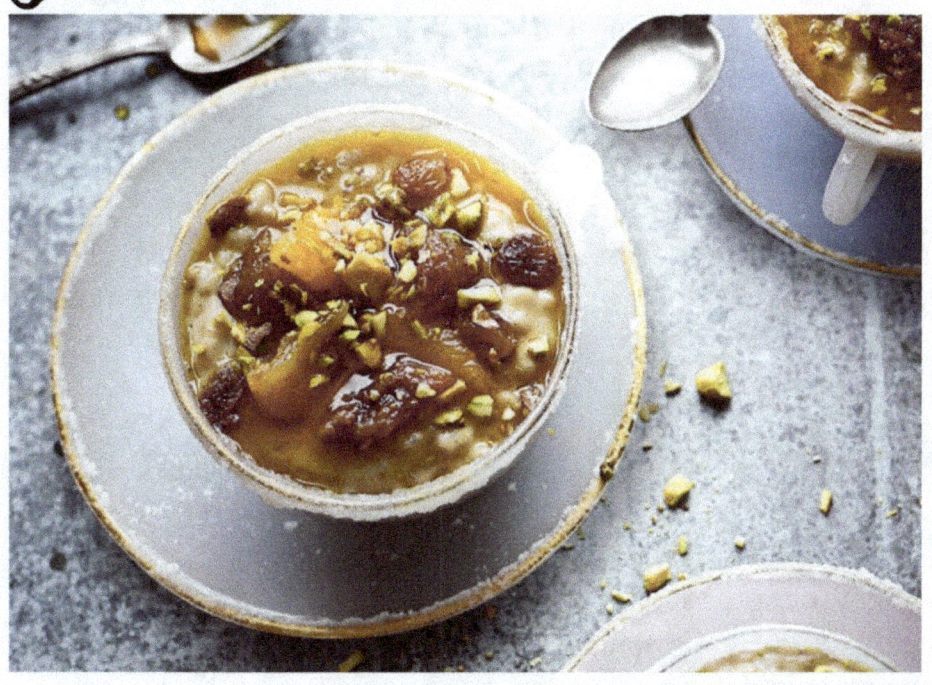

PREP
20 mins

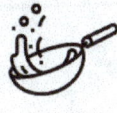
COOK
60 mins

SERVES
8-10

INGREDIENTS

1 litre whole milk (for a rich finish use gold top), plus extra – optional
400ml double cream
200g pudding rice
200g light brown soft sugar
150ml freshly brewed espresso (from a coffee machine – or use instant espresso powder)

2 tsp vanilla bean paste
150ml clear honey
Finely grated zest and juice 2 oranges
1 long cinnamon stick, or 2 short
400g mixed dried fruit, roughly chopped (we used sultanas, apricots and figs)
Handful unsalted pistachios, roughly chopped, to garnish

INSTRUCTIONS

Put all the rice pudding ingredients in a large heavy-based saucepan, bring to a gentle simmer and cook, stirring often, for 45-60 minutes until the rice is al dente. Keep an eye on it once it starts to thicken up as it can catch on the bottom of the pan. If the rice starts to dry out before it's ready, add extra milk. Meanwhile, put the honey, 200ml water, orange zest and juice in a pan over a medium heat. Add the cinnamon stick(s) and bring to a simmer. Add the fruit, reduce the heat and cook for 2-3 minutes, letting the mixture steam but not bubble. Turn off the heat and leave the fruit to steep until the rice is ready. Once the rice pudding is al dente – cooked but still with a little bite – turn off the heat, cover the top with a piece of cling film directly touching the surface to stop a skin forming, then leave it to rest. Drain the fruit in a sieve set over a bowl to catch the juices. Set the fruit aside and return the juices to the pan. Bring to the boil and reduce for around 10 minutes until syrupy. To serve, divide the rice pudding among bowls. Top with a couple of spoonfuls of the dried fruit, a generous drizzle of the syrup and a scattering of pistachios.

Strawberry Balsamic Sorbet

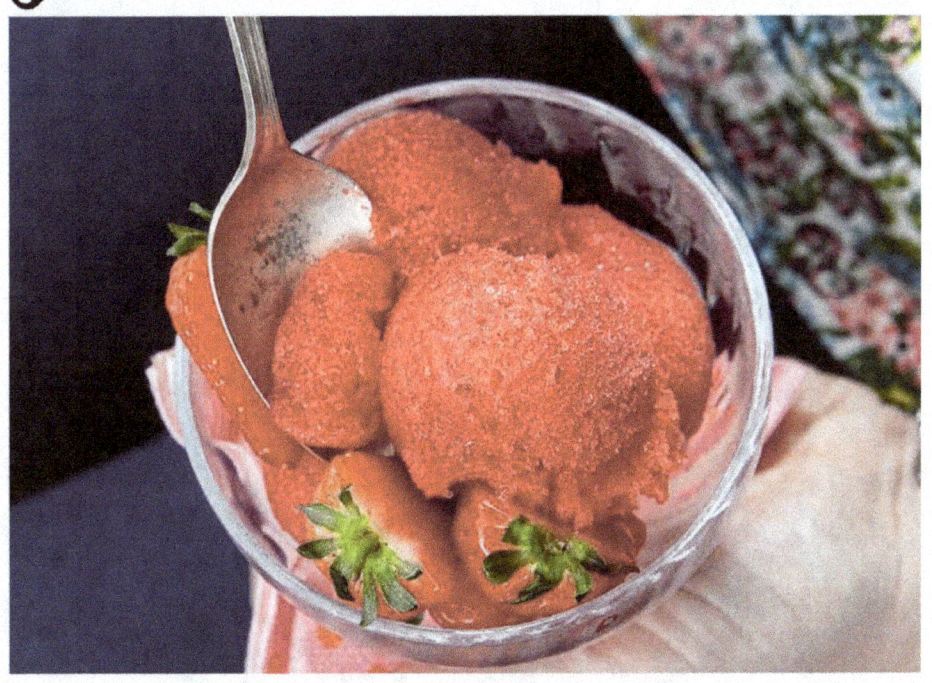

PREP
5 mins

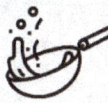
COOK
5 mins

SERVES
8-10

INGREDIENTS

Lemons 3, halved
Strawberries 900g (2lb), hulled and roughly chopped if large

Caster sugar 350g (12oz)
Balsamic vinegar 3–4 tsp

INSTRUCTIONS

Remove the pips from two of the lemon halves, roughly chop the halves and then blitz (flesh and skin) in a food processor with the sugar to make a sugary lemon paste.

Add the strawberries and whizz to a purée then stir in the juice from the other two lemons (approx. 100ml/3½fl oz) along with the balsamic vinegar.

Pour into a freezer-proof container, pushing the purée through a sieve to remove seeds if you prefer. Freeze for about 8 hours, taking it out after 3–4 hours, breaking it up and whizzing it in the food processor until smooth. Freeze again.

Serve scoops of sorbet with thin ginger biscuits or more fruit.

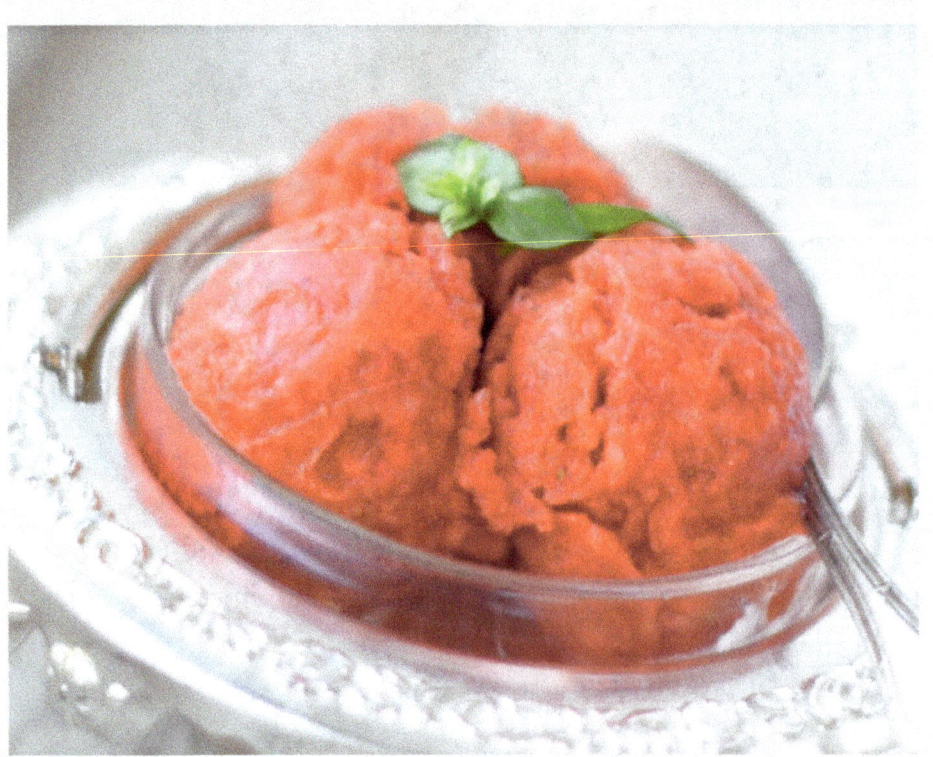

www.ingramcontent.com/pod-product-compliance
Lightning Source LLC
Chambersburg PA
CBHW071952210526
45479CB00003B/902